SOPHIA RISING

Awakening your sacred wisdom through yoga

TO MY MOM CISSIE WATSON—IN SUBVERSIVELY
FLANKING YOUR NATIVITY SCENE
WITH A MENORAH AND A BUDDHA YOU HELPED
BROADEN MY FAITH BEYOND ANY
ONE ICON—THANK YOU.

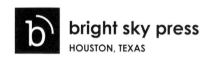

bright sky press
HOUSTON, TEXAS

2365 Rice Blvd., Suite 202
Houston, Texas 77005

10   9   8   7   6   5   4   3   2   1

Library of Congress Cataloging-in-Publication Data

Chilson, Monette, 1967-
Sophia rising : awakening your sacred wisdom through yoga / by Monette Chilson.
p. cm.
ISBN 978-1-936474-22-6
1. Yoga. 2. Christianity and yoga. I. Title.

B132.Y6C5833 2012
181'.45--dc23   2012023227

Editorial Direction, Lucy Herring Chambers
Editor, Eva Freeburn
Creative Direction, Ellen Peeples Cregan
Design, Marla Y. Garcia

Printed in Canada through Friesens

SOPHIA RISING

Awakening Your Sacred Wisdom Through Yoga

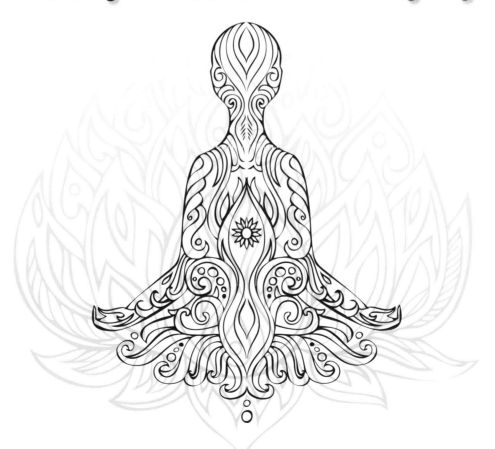

MONETTE CHILSON

table of contents

Author's Notes

Before we begin this journey together, I feel compelled to talk about the elephant in the room that I valiantly tried to avoid for many months. That elephant is the pronoun used in referencing God. I tried to avoid pronoun references to God altogether, but I eventually threw in the towel. It simply wasn't working. Sometimes I just needed one to keep the writing flowing and to imbue the expressions of divinity with an element of familiarity.

To that end, I took the image of God (among the many blessedly presented to us through scripture and other sacred writings) that currently spoke most strongly to me—Sophia (Greek for Wisdom)—and ran with that. Sophia is a female name, so I will use "she" and "her" when I find it necessary to interject a pronoun. I liken this approach to William P. Young's in his bestselling book, *The Shak,* in which God changes gender and form based on the character's need at that moment. If you stumble across a "she" or a "her" that sounds odd to your ears, know that I am expressing the pronoun that resonates most strongly with me at this point in my life. Also, if you are having difficulty with it, remember for just a moment, how many millions of times people have been subjected to a one-dimensional view of God as expressed through just one acceptable pronoun—he—for many thousands of years.

All Bible verses, unless otherwise indicated, have been cited from *The Inclusive Bible: The First Egalitarian Translation,* published by Sheed & Ward in 2007 and compiled by a group known as Priests for Equality. The Inclusive Bible translates the original Hebrew, Aramaic, and koiné Greek into richly poetic, non-sexist, and non-classist modern English.

Finally, a special note to the men who are reading this book (first and foremost to my husband whose encouragement prompted me to consciously invite men into this book and its dialog): I applaud you for "going there," for seeking out a holistic image of God for yourself, and for the women in your life. Whether you are a husband, a father, or the son of a woman, it is my hope that you will discover a long-discarded piece of your own spiritual DNA, while acquiring a perspective on God that will allow you to more fully comprehend the spiritual journey and obstacles of the women you love.

INTRODUCTION
seeking sophia

SHE IS THE LIGHT THAT SHINES FORTH FROM
EVERLASTING LIGHT,
THE FLAWLESS MIRROR OF THE DYNAMISM OF GOD
AND THE PERFECT IMAGE OF THE HOLY ONE'S
GOODNESS.
THOUGH ALONE OF HER KIND, SHE CAN DO ALL
THINGS;
THOUGH UNCHANGING, SHE RENEWS ALL THINGS;
GENERATION AFTER GENERATION SHE ENTERS INTO
HOLY SOULS
AND MAKES THEM FRIENDS OF GOD AND PROPHETS,
FOR GOD LOVES THE ONE
WHO FINDS A HOME IN WISDOM [SOPHIA].
SHE IS MORE BEAUTIFUL THAN THE SUN
AND MORE MAGNIFICENT THAN ALL THE STARS IN
THE SKY.
(WISDOM OF SOLOMON 7:26-8:1, THE INCLUSIVE BIBLE)

I would have stopped doodling mermaids and fallen off the worn oak pew in awed wonder had someone read me these verses as a child growing up in a small town Southern Baptist Church—especially if they had invoked the name of Sophia (Greek for Wisdom). Desperate to see myself reflected in my religion, I longed for someone to look beneath the patriarchal doctrine and dogma and show me that I was a part of the grand epic woven in the pages of the Bible. Someone to assure me that God wasn't the exclusively masculine being described from every pulpit I'd encountered in my young life.

I stumbled through my formative years, grasping at the good in my faith tradition, while grappling with the parts that didn't make sense to me. I couldn't shake the feeling that something was missing. I just didn't know where to find it. Often, I found myself going back to the same dry well looking for water. I faithfully played Mary every year in the church Christmas pageant, joined Girls in Action (like Baptist Girl Scouts), memorized famous women missionaries and studied their lives, looking for clues as to what inspired their faith. My freshman year in college I frequented the Baptist Student Union. I know now that doing the same thing over and over again and expecting different results is the definition of insanity. It was the only way I knew to live back then. I was searching for the spiritual essence of my faith, but I kept coming up empty-handed—or worse, disillusioned and dejected.

Luckily, God's ways are always more expansive than mine. I was slowly drawn along a path that makes sense in retrospect, one that honored some inner wisdom regarding my physical and spiritual self. I was the oddball that asked for a juicer for Christmas one year in high school. Then I stopped eating meat after writing a paper on vegetarianism my sophomore year in college. I was always intrigued by yoga and finally began practicing a few years out of school. Through this progression, I learned to be true to myself—the person God was calling me to be—even when it went against the grain of my Southern upbringing.

I didn't know that my yoga practice would be the antidote to the unrest I felt with my religious life. I had no idea the missing piece of practical spiritual wisdom I'd been seeking would appear as I sat on a mat in an incense-filled room listening to unfamiliar words chanted in Eastern

10

tongues. How strange it felt to have finally found my spiritual home while simultaneously fearing I was betraying my faith tradition.

On my mat I felt the part of God that had eluded me for years. God flowed into me on my breath, moved through my limbs and settled into my heart center at the end of my practice. Suddenly God was free to be God, or rather I was freed to experience God without the inferences of maleness. It took me a while to recognize God in this new guise. There were no robes, crosses, or religious icons to tip me off. I could see myself reflected in this new divine vision.

While today I intuitively interpret that feeling as God at work in me, back then I didn't know what to make of it. I knew it felt spiritual, but I had no way to explain this newfound spirituality or to integrate it into my religious beliefs. For a while, it worked because I had put religion on hold during my post-college twenty-something years. I simply buried my fears about yoga being contrary to the Christianity of my youth. My yogic spirituality sustained me, while I pointedly avoided organized religion. When my husband and I became parents and decided to go back to church in our thirties, I began the process of reconciling the two.

First I tried making my yoga Christian. I thought it quite clever to find Bible verses to accompany my favorite poses. For example, I used Psalm 45:3-4, "Strap your sword to your side, warrior! Accept praise! Accept due honor! Ride majestically! Ride triumphantly! Ride on the side of truth! Ride for the righteous meek," to sanctify warrior pose. I had corresponding verses for bow pose, child's pose, mountain pose, and others. I convinced myself that if I read Bible verses with my poses, they would be redeemed. That my faith and my practice would become one. I was bridging the chasm with holy words.

I developed and taught a class using this approach. We opened by meditating to a folksy version of the classic Christian hymn *Be Thou My Vision* and ended by listening to my good friend Robbie Seay's *Breathe Peace* in *savasana* (still a favorite of mine). In between, we did yoga poses to a litany of Bible verses I had carefully chosen as the soundtrack to our practice. While this Christianized yoga was a valuable stepping stone for me, it ultimately felt contrived—like I was trying to make both yoga and Christianity something they weren't. I had yet to realize that the chasm

I was attempting to bridge didn't exist. The two weren't as spiritually incompatible as I had been led to believe.

I knew that the sacred source I encountered on my yoga mat was not male. In fact, it felt distinctly feminine to me. Was it because I was finally seeing myself mirrored in God? Or was there, legitimately, a female side of God that existed in my faith tradition? How could this have been overlooked or ignored by so many? And why did I find her here in my yoga practice instead of in church? Did I dare to explore this unorthodox view I was beginning to espouse?

It was these questions that ultimately set in motion the research that culminated in this book. It was this quest that led me to Sophia and enabled me to practice both yoga and Christianity without internal conflict or angst. The answers I found made me whole again. It is my fervent hope that my experience will light the way for others out there looking for their own answers and seeking to integrate their yogic and religious lives.

Though we may be on similar trajectories, each of our paths is our own. Sophia was the key to my spiritual reconciliation. Her role in your journey may be significant or peripheral. In either case, you owe it to yourself to meet her.

Greek for wisdom, Sophia surfaces repeatedly in both the Christian and Hebrew[1] scriptures, yet her identity remains unclear. Some see Sophia as a deity in her own right, others see her as representing the Bride of Christ (Revelation 19), others as a feminine aspect of God representing wisdom (Proverbs 8 and 9), and still others as a theological concept regarding the wisdom of God. Sophia, by her very nature, defies definition, allowing us to revel in the mystery that surrounds her.

She is there within each and every one of us—male and female—whether we choose to embrace or deny her existence. She is the Holy Spirit. She is the breath we breathe. She is God-given, not something women dreamt up to make us feel better about being left out of all the starring roles in the Bible. The truth is, we weren't left out. Sophia was there all along, beckoning to us—right along with Jesus. And it's not just

---

1   The Jewish faith would, obviously, use the Hebrew translation of Wisdom rather than the Greek word Sophia. Because of its nuances, you might find Wisdom expressed as khokhma (wisdom), bina (understanding), da'at (knowledge) or tvuna (another word for understanding).

women who were short-changed in the masculinization of God. Men, too, long to be able to experience God holistically, to acknowledge and rest in the feminine side of God.

Most of us will pay lip service to the fact that God transcends gender, but our experience—because of the stigma associated with the feminine divine in Western religions—does not include prayers, images, or words that let us express this truth. Whether the aversion to referring to God in feminine terms stems from patriarchal roots, a desire by early Christians to separate themselves from Goddess worship or to differentiate themselves from Gnostic communities, the result has been a severing of the sacred feminine that has silenced voices that would pray to God our Mother. Sophia embodies those missing pieces, giving us the prayers, images and words we need to complete our limited human perspective on who God is—and who God wants to be—in our lives.

Bringing that awareness of Sophia into focus is a function of being, rather than doing. It is passive, not active, and it requires us to back off and surrender to that voice that is whispering to us even when our internal dialog drowns it out. So how do we listen to a voice we can't hear? There are many ways to attune ourselves to divine utterances. The commonality of all these paths lies in the contemplative stance they require and deep spiritual connection they illicit. In psychological parlance, an introverted practice is needed to balance the extroverted world in which we live.

Yoga, in its fullness (not just its poses), can provide spiritual seekers with the tools they need to start hearing that sacred song they've been missing. By providing a space devoid of any pre-programmed liturgy, sermons or psalms, they allow us to sit with God. To move with God. Even to chant melodious syllables full of life force to God. Finally, to discover God.

When we sit in a church pew (regardless of the religion), we are surrounded by others' perceptions of God, both visual and spoken. When we sit on our yoga mat, we are carving out space for our own spiritual life to coalesce, creating our inner sanctuaries, and opening ourselves up to God's presence—untainted and unfiltered by religious precepts. Yoga doesn't create the sacred. It merely reveals it in many beautiful ways.

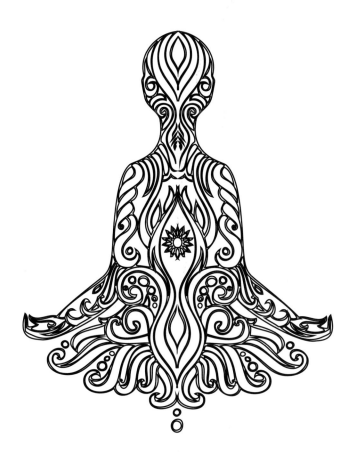

CHAPTER I

The Uniting Force of Yoga

YOGA IS A UNITING FORCE ON SO MANY LEVELS. THE VERY ROOT OF THE WORD MEANS "UNION." THAT UNITY MANIFESTS ITSELF IN DIFFERENT WAYS DEPENDING ON THE PERSON PRACTICING IT, THE FAITH OR INTENTION BEHIND THE PRACTICE, AND THE SPECIFIC NEEDS OF THE PRACTITIONER AT THAT MOMENT. SERVING AS A TOUCHPOINT—A WELLSPRING—THROUGH TIMES OF DOUBT, TIMES OF FAITH, TIMES OF OVERWHELMING SORROW, AND TIMES OF REJOICING IN GOD'S AMAZING ABUNDANCE, YOGA IS A POWERFUL TOOL FOR HEALING. ONE THAT IS OFTEN MISUNDERSTOOD.

As a Christian, I am often saddened by the divisive rhetoric and actions that some invoke in the name of Christianity, and yoga feels like an antidote to that. Religions have been twisted to meet cultural needs since the dawn of time, and Christianity is no exception. One unknown commentator noted, "The Jews tried to keep Christ contained within their law, while the Greeks sought to turn Him into a philosophy; the Romans made of Him an empire; the Europeans reduced Him to a culture, and we Americans have made a business of Him."

A pastor friend of mine dances around the title of "pastor" or "preacher" when he meets new people. Instead, he refers to his other roles as author and speaker—not because he is ashamed of what he does. To the contrary, he has realized that the baggage that comes with the word pastor—in the Christian sense as it's often interpreted within our postmodern culture—instantly shuts down authentic dialog with many of them. These people don't want to hear about the Jesus that has been carefully packaged to "sell" to Americans.

Likewise, putting a spiritual system as complex as yoga into a box that works for the churched masses—renaming its poses—and changing it just enough to make it feel Christian—is not the answer. On the path I have chosen, yoga and Christianity are intertwined, complementing each other and bringing new depth to my spirituality. Neither yoga nor Christianity needs to be altered or stifled to fit within the confines of the other. I know many others walk this path and that, perhaps, they have felt they've walked it alone. Or that there was no path at all in this spiritual wilderness.

Sometimes I try to illuminate this path by referring to "Jesus," rather than "Christianity." Jesus, after all, represents the purest form of Christianity, the one part of this diverse, global religion that brings us all together. Even non-Christians respect Jesus as a prophet, a good and wise man who made a profound impact on the world.

Mahatma Ghandi, a practicing Hindu and one of history's greatest advocates for peace, described Jesus as "a man who was completely innocent, offered himself as a sacrifice for the good of others, including his enemies, and became the ransom of the world. It was a perfect act." Committed atheist and acclaimed science fiction writer H.G. Wells expressed his views on Jesus, saying, "I am an historian, I am not a believer, but I must confess as an historian that this penniless preacher from Nazareth is irrevocably the very center of history. Jesus Christ is easily the most dominant figure in all history." ⅄

Albert Einstein summed up the effect of Jesus in his statement: "As a child I received instruction both in the Bible and in the Talmud. I am a Jew, but I am enthralled by the luminous figure of the Nazarene.... No one can read the Gospels without feeling the actual presence of Jesus. His personality pulsates in every word. No myth is filled with such life." Quite a testament from those who are firm non-believers in the Jesus of the Christian faith.

Christians, of course, recognize Jesus on an even deeper level—as the Christ, the Messiah, that came to save us through the union of humanity and divinity. For Christians who practice yoga, this becomes a powerful symbol for us as we try to unite the humanity and divinity within each of us. One simple way of representing this unity with the physical body is through *anjali mudra*—a common yogic hand gesture in which the palms are placed together, typically just under the heart (anatomically, directly below the middle of the breastbone). In this *mudra*, often used to open and close a yoga class, one hand represents the higher, spiritual nature, while the other represents the worldly self. By combining the two, we acknowledge this dichotomy that exists within each of us and attempt to integrate the two sides from within. For many Christians, Jesus is a natural focus of meditation on this core spiritual endeavor as he embodies a perfect fusion of the two.

My own spiritual quest has taught me that yoga isn't about discovering the obvious truths in life. It is about going within and discovering the sublime make-up of our own souls, our own unique place in this world, and our own God-given purpose. Sophia is the aspect of God that perfectly embodies that journey of discovery for me. She is not well-known. In fact, She is not even recognized by many. But that's OK. God isn't into fame and fortune. God doesn't care who knows your name. I hear Sophia when I breathe and when I move, and so it only seemed fitting that she be my focus.

YOGA AS A TOOL FOR HEALING GENDER WOUNDS

Yoga's power to heal deep inner divides has been particularly helpful to me. As a woman, I have tried to live out my faith in a Christian tradition in which even the most enlightened of Christian bodies are building their communities on the foundation of a text which was translated by men for a society which validated men's roles. Women's roles have been relegated to the sidebars of history and to the margins of the Biblical stories. I say this not to diminish the authority of the Bible, but to put its journey—from God's unblemished wellspring of wisdom into the book that sits in our church pews today—into perspective. This assertion may sound subjective, but let's look at a simple linguistic analysis of the Bible's New International Version, often cited as the most popular translation.

Appearance of the word (NIV):

| **Mother:** 312 | **Her:** 1,595 | **Hers:** 46 |
| **Father:** 1,374 | **Him:** 4,573 | **His:** 5,386 |

More than seventy-five percent of all references to parental roles are paternal, rather than maternal. Similarly, in a broader context, the male pronoun "him" is used nearly three times as often as its female counter-part "her." In the most staggering contrast, when the concept of posses-sion is brought into the picture, "hers" is used a mere forty-six times in the entire Bible. This includes forms of the word like "herself," while "his"—the equivalent male possessive form and its variations—is used 5,386 times. Linguistically speaking, more than ninety-nine percent of the Bible's ownership is rooted in masculine language, thus in masculine imagery. For every one time we read about something being "hers" in the Bible, we will read 117 references to "his" possessions, "his" attributes, "his" desires—in essence, to "his" story (also known as "history"). How much more difficult does that language make it for women to own their own faith?

This linguistic discrepancy is not consistent with God's message to us. God's message, like all aspects of God, is pure and untainted—free of cor-ruption of any kind. The message, as necessitated by the societal norms of the period, was transcribed by men, edited by men, and finally, trans-lated from one language to another by men. God is infallible. Men are not. Neither are women, but if we'd been included in the conversation, at least there would have been some diversity in the perspectives and baggage brought to the table.

When I read the Bible, I am often overwhelmed and unable to iden-
tify with its imbalanced gender perspective. I become weary of hearing
about the God of Abraham, Isaac, and Jacob and wonder where the God
of Sarah, Rebekah, and Rachel was through it all. I love the lessons given to
us by the Desert Fathers, but I can't help wondering about what wisdom
the Desert Mothers would have imparted had their voices been recorded.
The Bible's message speaks to me, but the exclusively masculine language
and perspective gets in the way. In my heart of hearts I know that our
understanding of God is not intended to be more "his" than "hers," or
vice versa. God's love and the stories that tell of that love are intended to
speak to humanity—male and female. Genesis 1:27 says, "Humankind was
created as God's reflection: in the divine image God created them; female
and male, God made them." Contemplative author and speaker Richard
Rohr points out, "That must mean there are two major manifestations of
the divine image." We have been fed plentiful amounts of one of those
images while being deprived, to the point of starvation, of the other.

As a lover of words who understands the power they have over us—
especially the sacred words of God—I do believe that the disparity is too
great for us not to be affected by it. We are, after all, mere humans. We are
not endowed with God's ability to transcend such things and filter through
the messenger's humanity to get directly to the heart of the message.

This imbalance in gender representation cannot help but create an internal divide—though often denied—for women who attempt to base
their lives on its truths. The process is insidious, though well intentioned.
We hear God referred to as "He" so many times. We are taught to pray to
"Our Father who art in heaven," but not to God our Mother.

If we are in a "progressive" Christian church, we may hear an occasional
reference to God's "feminine" (i.e., nurturing) qualities, but we will almost
never learn that God's very wisdom is called by the feminine name "Sophia"
in the Bible. There are exceptions, of course—pastors who feel led to address the confusion surrounding Sophia from their pulpits. I happened upon
a sermon online, by Reverend James Roghair to the First Congregational
Church of Evanston, Illinois, in 2006. Roghair's sermon, based on an alternate lectionary reading from the Wisdom of Solomon, looks at Sophia
from a Biblical and historical standpoint and concludes that Sophia is "not

a goddess, but a way of recognizing God in us." Testifying to the courage it took to preach such a sermon, Roghair opens with this disclaimer: "I hope that reading this Deuterocanonical passage has not shocked your sensibilities. Although I know it would be highly offensive to some, I hope most of you won't mind. And I promise I won't do it often."

Why are we so very afraid of seeing God as female? Or even of acknowledging the female aspects of God? The entrenched idea that God is male is not Biblical. The Bible is clear on the fact that God is genderless, yet we continue to use male pronouns exclusively when referring to God. Sophia has become my way of accessing all that God intended in the vibrantly painted epic saga that is the Bible. Yoga has become my way of connecting with God directly, unmediated by religion.

This idea that God is male inevitably spills over into other aspects of religious life, often subjugating the role of women to that of men in both public and private realms. I can choose to expend negative energy fighting that system within settings where the prejudices still exist, or I can opt to worship in communities where those limitations don't exist and redirect my energy into positive channels through yoga and meditation. These tools—though outside the traditional Christian toolbox—provide me with a way to access God without any external projections of gender. It simply becomes a non-issue when it's just me and God moving, breathing, and journeying together. God does not have to conform to labels like "Father" or "Lord." When I'm doing yoga, God just "is"—much like in Exodus 3:14 when God declares, "I AM who I AM" (NIV).

The *Inclusive Bible* translates God's defining proclamation as, "I AM that I AM." God transcends even the concept of "who-ness." Getting beyond the quest for God's identity and experiencing the pureness of "I AM"— divine wholeness—ultimately led me to live more peacefully.

YOGA AS A BRIDGE BETWEEN FAITHS & CULTURES

I have chosen to live as a Christian. Am I convinced that Christianity is the only way to commune with God? The only way to be saved from eternal damnation? No. I have found that statement causes some Christians much consternation. It is simply not my place to judge such things. It is my place to love God with all my heart, my soul, and all my strength (Deuteronomy

6:5). It is also my job to love my neighbors and even my enemies (Matthew 5:44). It is God's job, in her infinite wisdom, to decide how all the stuff of the afterlife plays out. Matthew 6:34, which we will look at in depth a little later, really says it better than I can: "Enough of worrying about tomorrow! Let tomorrow take care of itself. Today has troubles enough of its own." Living faithfully is definitely a large enough task for me. I will let God be the judge of how well I am—and the rest of the world is—doing.

Yoga becomes a bridge between faiths and cultures in the simplest of ways—by recognizing that God lives in each of us. The standard finale of yoga classes across the globe is "*namaste.*" This Sanskrit word means, "I see the Light in you, and I honor it." It is typically said with hands in the *anjali mudra*—prayer position—at the heart and with a slight bow of the head. Light is somewhat ambiguous (and the capitalization is mine), but to me, it clearly says God. It doesn't discriminate or limit the presence of God to those of a specific religion or belief system, as in, "I see the Light in you and honor it *if* you are the same religion that I am." It is physical embodiment of the bumper sticker wisdom, "God Bless Everyone—No Exceptions."

The majority of the people who have expressed their concerns to me about yoga being incompatible with their faith list the fact that yoga talks about the God within each of us as their biggest issue. They mistakenly think this is deifying humanity. Instead, it is actually honoring that place in each of us where God dwells. Christians express this concept as being filled with the Holy Spirit. In Judaism, *Shekhinah* (whose root means "dwelling") expresses the indwelling of God. Interestingly, *Shekhinah* is the only of God's principle names that is grammatically feminine in the Hebrew language. Its Arabic counterpart, *Sakina,* is found in the Qur'an.

When I try to explain this distinction, they generally shake their head and say something like, "Yes, yes, I know about the Holy Spirit. Of course I remember that God dwells in me that way, but this—this is something different. Yoga is talking about some other God, and it says that God lives inside *everybody*!" When I still appear unoffended by this obvious heresy, they either give up and label me one of those New Age types, or they are intrigued by the fact that I tolerate—even more startling, that I embrace—this assertion that God lives in all of us.

Going back to the source of Christian wisdom—to the scriptures—

Romans 8:11 says, "If the Spirit of the One who raised Jesus from the dead, dwell in you, then the One who raised Christ from the dead will also bring your mortal bodies to life through the Spirit dwelling in you." After reading that passage, I am drawn back to the idea that it is not my job to decide "if the Spirit of the One who resurrected Jesus lives inside" anyone other than myself.

If I were to define yoga in Biblical terms, "bringing this mortal body to life through the Spirit dwelling within" is a pretty good description of how yoga works. I have tried all kinds of yoga classes and I can honestly say that explicitly Christian yoga classes have not been the most moving for me. Since I've brought up the whole questionable concept of bumper sticker wisdom, let's go back to a much over-used one, "What would Jesus do?" Would he go to the temple and do yoga only with the high-ranking Jews of the day? Or would we be more likely to find him in the "bad" part of town, blanket spread out amongst the beggars and the homeless, chanting blessings to the poor while he taught the children how to move and breathe in life—regardless of the squalor surrounding them?

This is yoga to me—faiths coming together, our mats touching, our lives overlapping, ancient wisdom reaching across time and space to touch each person in a unique way—in the exact way each needs to be met on that day and in that moment. I am quite certain that the one doing the reaching is God—not *my* God or *your* God. Just God. Namaste.

YOGA AS A HOLISTIC SPIRITUAL EXPERIENCE

I am continually reminded that yoga is a metaphor for life, and I delight in coming up with monikers that represent yoga's role in my life at any given moment. One of my favorites is "the great excavator." If I have an issue—physical, mental, or spiritual—that I am unaware of or in denial about, Sophia, in her wisdom, will use my yoga practice to dig it up from its hidden depths and expose it. If I am paying attention, she will teach me things about myself that I wouldn't otherwise know. If I act on that knowledge, it is almost always transformative. While many of these specific lessons will be covered in Chapter 4 (Lessons from the Mat), I want to introduce the concept here because it is at the core of what Sophia does for me through my yoga.

Yoga is a holistic experience. It involves the whole self. As I deeply work my body, my mind is enlightened and my spirit touched in mysterious ways. It is the unity of the body, mind, and spirit that makes yoga so powerful. For Christians, it is a metaphorical way to move deeper into the trinitarian concept that is the basis of our faith.

Body... Yoga informs us about our body and, in the process, teaches us spiritual lessons. Recently, I went into class feeling just fine, ready to move through whatever my teacher had for us that day. Just thirty minutes into the hour and a half class I began to feel nauseated, hot and lightheaded. I tried to push through for a few minutes but then stopped in mid-pose to rest. My highly intuitive teacher came over and checked in with me. She asked if I had been sick this week. I said, "No, but my kids have."

She noted that in the past couple of weeks, many people had experienced this feeling after being exposed to circulating viral strains. I hadn't even exhibited any symptoms of sickness prior to class. My conscious mind did not know there was a virus floating around somewhere in my body. When my yoga practice went to work from the inside out, the lurking virus showed up and knocked me out.

The good news is that it came out. That's what you want to happen. You don't want sickness and disease lurking, hidden within your body. You want to move them out to be expunged.

My natural inclination was to push through and let it all out! But, as in so many areas of my life, I needed to simply be gentle with myself and respect that I was not well. I didn't need to label my self "sick" or "weak." I just needed to say that my body was telling me that I needed to rest.

My yoga at that moment was to learn to respect my body's needs and simply rest. So, in the middle of a band of mighty warriors, I lay down in a restorative pose, lying back on a bolster and honored my body's unique needs in that particular space and time. I did a variety of restorative poses for the rest of the class, and by the time it was over, I felt like I had done some much-needed physical healing that I wouldn't have known I needed to do had I not come to class that morning.

Mind... The concept of our physical body needing time to recover is widely accepted in our culture. Even body builders follow a regime that gives each muscle group every other day off. But the idea of a respite for our ever-busy minds is foreign to most of us. In the periods of the day that I consider my "downtime," I still don't turn off my mind—not really. I read. I write. I check emails. I look something up on the web. I make phone calls. All these tasks can be done from my favorite comfy chair at Starbucks. But while my body is chilling, the wheels in my mind are whirring.

The mind is a powerful thing. We focus on building strength in our bodies through yoga, but we are strengthening our minds as much as we are our bodies. We are training the mind to be still.

Often I can make it through an *asana* (posture) with unwavering focus because I am focusing on something specific—an action to be accomplished, constructive work to be done. This is familiar and comfortable turf for me. Making it through the period of *savasana* (resting pose or corpse pose) at the end of class is a much tougher challenge for my mind. At that point the "work" of the class is over, as we define "work" in our culture. There is nothing to be accomplished. There is no doing left to do, only "being" left to be.

It's a true challenge for my mind to remain still in the absence of a task. The lack of a task does not stop my mind from trying. "No task to be done now?" quips my mind. "No problem! I'll start working on those tasks that need to be done later today—even get a head start on tomorrow!" When I can remain in the moment, I experience peace like no other. It feels like I'm living out my favorite scripture, "Be still and know that I am God" (Psalm 46:10). In eight words, this verse manages to sum up a way of life I wish I could lead—not just for minutes during my yoga practice—but day in and day out.

Spirit... Yoga has taught me that the true beauty of spirituality is found in the subtleties—in the things that at first blush are not apparent. They emerge only when we are ready for them, much as Sophia appeared to me from the very same text I'd read all my life. I am reminded of the old Zen proverb, "When the student is ready, the teacher will come." Whenever I get to a point of readiness for a particular lesson, I find Sophia there, sitting on my yoga mat, ready to teach me. I must simply be present. The present is just that—a present, a gift to be treasured, opened and savored each and every moment of our lives. If we are not in the present, we are by default in the past or the future. When I have defected from the present, I am not on the path that Sophia has so lovingly mapped out for me. I am missing whatever is actually happening in my life, and there is no backtracking to recapture the time I have given over to lamenting what has already happened or fretting about what is yet to come.

This principal of living in the moment often gets thrown under the umbrella of New Age spirituality. What many people consider New Age mumbo jumbo actually has very strong biblical roots. Jesus was a very deep guy. He didn't spell many things out or provide us with ten steps to joyful living. What he did was tell stories—and boy could he spin a yarn. The difficulty with that particular form of literary technique—and the beauty of it—is that it leaves a lot of the work up to us. We listen to a parable. We roll it around on our tongues like a new wine we are tasting, sensing the subtle flavors that emerge as it moves over our palate and down our throats. Jesus wanted us to do this. His words were designed to be savored.

The problem arises when we try to take shortcuts. Many of us, at some point in our academic lives, have tried the CliffsNotes approach to a great literary work. And many of us have done it with Jesus' stories, too. We have accepted the simplified version we first learned in the Sunday school lessons of our childhoods. Sure, we get the basic facts. We hear how someone else interpreted the master's eloquent prose, but we miss out on the magic. We miss the beauty. Our experience ceases to be personally moving and becomes just another academic exercise.

We hear passages preached on and written about. We let other people interpret God's words for us. Just as if we had used the CliffsNotes, we miss the point. There really are CliffsNotes for the Bible. On the cover is a timer emblazoned with the words, "Fast, Proven, Trusted." The Bible is not designed for speed-reading. God is not giving us extra points for getting through it faster than the next guy. Proven? God's word is about faith, not proof. And trusted? Well, let's just say I'd be in sad shape if I trusted the publishers of CliffsNotes more than I trusted God.

Jesus, in his flowing, round-about way, was pointing us to the importance of many truths that we may not be fully or personally grasping if we let other people interpret for us. One of these truths has become glaringly clear to me as I practice yoga and experience that deep stillness and communion with Sophia. It is the profound importance of keeping myself in the now, so that she can work in me and through me. After grasping that spiritual concept through my yoga practice, I was able to see that the words of Jesus were pointing to it all along. I was not taking the words in deeply enough. I was just reading them at a superficial level.

I love to read the works of Eckhart Tolle again and again. He picks up on this limiting interpretation of scripture in his book *The Power of Now*, throughout which he quotes Jesus, along with other spiritual leaders. He puts scripture I had been exposed to all my life into a whole new context. He never actually gives verses (or even books of the Bible) for the passages he quotes. Often, it is just a thought or phrase attributed to Jesus. I like the open-endedness of that approach. It led me to seek out the actual passages and read them for myself. Seeking a richer context still, I read them in several different translations. They began to open up to me in whole new ways.

Sophia uses my yoga practice to blessedly entangle body, mind and spirit. An awakening in one realm starts a domino effect that brings a similar awakening in the others. I experience something physically in yoga class that leads me to explore an idea intellectually or spiritually, and then it is finally integrated as it completes its journey through all three realms.

It creates a circle within me where God is the Alpha and Omega, and there is no end to the wisdom that I can absorb if I can keep myself open on all three fronts. I consider this the divine wisdom—embodied as Sophia—that God wants to impart to me, if only I will slow down enough to hear it, to feel it, and to live it.

YOGA AS PATH TO THE PURE, UNMITIGATED DIVINE

Seeing ourselves as the primary authors of our own faith does not discount the need for a religious foundation and a faith community. The spiritual leaders within those communities can speak into our lives by reminding us to take responsibility for our own spiritual lives. If we live responsibly through tasks like balancing our checkbooks, giving philanthropically, and researching all things health-related, then how can we abdicate the responsibility for the most important aspect of our lives, our spiritual livelihood? We can't let others dictate our experience with God.

A friend of mine describes this as *"shoulding* on ourselves." We try to convince ourselves that we believe what we *should* believe. We attempt to mold our experiences to what we are told they *should* be. We question our responses that are not what we think they *should* be.

Every time you hear that voice in your head telling you that you *should* be something... do something... think something that doesn't ring true to you, a red flag is waving. Sure, we all have very real responsibilities—things we truly need to do and obligations to which we have committed ourselves. But the vast majority of the time, the *shoulds* bouncing around in my head are not real *shoulds* but merely impersonators that distract me from focusing on the moment at hand and what Sophia wants for me in that moment.

I was always taught that the core of the Bible verses on living in the moment were about not worrying and trusting in God. But there was a deeper, more profound meaning that I wasn't getting. God always wants more for us than we can imagine. God doesn't just want to see us *give up worrying* about tomorrow but wants us to *fully embrace* today. The difference may seem like semantics, but it is equivalent to the difference between waiting for the Kingdom of God in the afterlife and creating it here on Earth. The first scenario leads to a life of tolerance and waiting—a life of mediocrity—while the second leads to a life of God's fullness *now*, with the promise that inner joy will remain regardless of the state of your physical body.

Let's take a look at what scripture says:

> All this time and money wasted on fashion—do you think it makes that much difference? Instead of looking at the fashions, walk out into the fields and look at the wildflowers. They never primp or shop, but have you ever seen color and design quite like it? The ten best-dressed men and women in the country look shabby alongside them. If God gives such attention to the appearance of wildflowers—most of which are never even seen—don't you think he'll attend to you, take pride in you, do his best for you? What I'm trying to do here is to get you to relax, to not be so preoccupied with getting, so you can respond to God's giving (Matthew 6:28-30, The Message).

This modern translation homes in on a phenomenon to which all of us in our media saturated culture can, unfortunately, relate—comparing ourselves to the men and women on those best-dressed lists. I love the thought that they look shabby compared to the simple beauty of the wildflowers that God created and placed out in the middle of nowhere. Out of the limelight, just for the sake of creation, whether anyone ever sees them or not. That is the part of the verse that illustrates so beautifully why we shouldn't fret and worry about our needs being met.

My favorite part, the real meat of that section that gives us the impetus for doing things differently, is the part about not being so preoccupied with getting that we miss the opportunity to respond to God's giving. Truly, I know from experience that it is possible to be so busy promoting our own agendas that we miss the beauty God has already placed right in front of us. It's like the old saying about taking time to smell the roses. We can get so busy rushing to wherever it is we've decided we "should" go, that we don't even see the roses, much less take time to smell them. One of my favorite ways of reconnecting when I'm feeling like I need some grounding is to walk through our yard and look for flowers that have appeared since my last stroll. I can't take credit for growing those beautiful blooms (that would be my green-thumbed husband), but I can soak in their simple beauty and be grateful for their presence. Sometimes I even grab my camera and snap a few pictures to pull out during those winter months when the blooms are not as plentiful.

The importance of being in the "now" comes up again in the Gospel of Luke when Jesus replies to a man who wants to say goodbye to his family before leaving to follow him, "Whoever puts a hand on the plow but keeps looking back is unfit for the reign of God" (Luke 9:62). Statements like this have convinced me that the Bible is written primarily in metaphor and parables. What we know of Jesus' character does not lead us to believe he would literally forbid someone from going back to say goodbye to his mother or father before embarking on trip to spread the Gospel. So, what does it mean?

The beauty of the Bible is that the meaning is left up to the interpretation of the reader. I am immediately wary of anyone who is absolutely certain of the meaning of each of Jesus' divine utterances. Jesus is clearly not giving us a step-by-step plan for salvation but instead is painting a picture whose beauty surpasses that of any of the great masters. He is not advocating that we abandon our families when we choose to follow him. And I can't imagine that he really cares whether we steal a backwards glance when and if we ever happen to find ourselves behind a plow.

What I believe he does care about is that we not put our pursuit of the world (even our earthly families who live in it) before our pursuit of God. Much of our purpose here on earth is to stay focused on the divine at work in our lives that is speaking to our souls—at this moment. If we are looking behind us as we plow, we might just miss what God has so lovingly sown in the row right in front of us.

The Message translation has a different flavor, going back to the idea that living in the moment allows us to experience God's kingdom, grace, and beauty now instead of in an afterlife: "No procrastination. No backward looks. You can't put God's kingdom off till tomorrow. Seize the day."

One of my favorite singers, Carolyn Arends, articulates this idea better than I could.

Well one thing I've noticed, wherever I wander
Everyone's got a dream he can follow or squander
You can do what you will with the days you are given
I'm trying to spend mine on the business of living
So I'm singing my songs off of any old stage
You can laugh if you want, I'll still say
Seize the day, seize whatever you can
'Cause life slips away just like hourglass sand
Seize the day, pray for grace from God's hand
Then nothing will stand in your way
Seize the day.

CAROLYN ARENDS "SEIZE THE DAY"
© 1995 SUNDAY SHOES MUSIC (ASCAP)

It is through this seizing of the day that we are able to experience "God with us" *now*—at this very moment, in this very life (*Emmanuel,* Hebrew for Christ). It is this action that paves each of our unique paths to the pure unmitigated divine. I firmly believe that there are many routes to God. It feels presumptuous to think that a being as all-encompassing as God could be restricted to just one path. Yoga is mine, and Sophia is my guide.

CHAPTER 2

The Heart of Yoga

ACCORDING TO B.K.S. IYENGAR, WIDELY REGARDED AS THE FATHER OF MODERN YOGA, THE WORD "YOGA," DERIVED FROM THE SANSKRIT ROOT "YUJ," MEANS TO BIND, JOIN, ATTACH AND YOKE, TO DIRECT AND CONCENTRATE ONE'S ATTENTION ON, TO USE AND APPLY. THIS DEFINITION BEGS THE QUESTIONS, "BIND, YOKE AND ATTACH TO WHAT?" "DIRECT AND CONCENTRATE OUR ATTENTION ON WHAT?" "WHAT ARE WE USING AND APPLYING?" IF WE DIG DEEPER INTO THE ROOTS OF THE WORD, WE DISCOVER IT ALSO MEANS UNION OR COMMUNION AND HAS BEEN DESCRIBED AS THE TRUE UNION OF OUR WILL WITH THE WILL OF GOD. EVEN WHEN USED IN NON-SPIRITUAL CONTEXTS, THE WORD YOGA ALWAYS REFERS TO SOME TYPE OF UNION. FOR EXAMPLE, IN ASTRONOMY IT REFERS TO A CONJUNCTION (UNION) OF PLANETS.

This core idea of unity is what makes yoga such a powerful tool for transformation. What we are ultimately using and applying is the wisdom that God has already planted in each of our souls. Yoga becomes a tool we can use to slowly chip away at the wall—made up of defenses, coping mechanisms, misguided ideas about ourselves, our world and our God—that encircles that divine spark, the holiest of spirits, that dwells in the core of our being.

Sometimes I wonder if this deeper meaning of yoga—the real yoga—has gotten lost in the shuffle of Westernized power yoga—buried under piles of chic yoga clothing, hemp mats, designer yoga bags, cork blocks and videos "starring" yoga icons.

By taking the spirit out of yoga, we have taken the life out of it, making this ancient system just another form of exercise for those questing after longer lives, more flexible bodies, and a way to escape from the rat race for a few moments. There is nothing inherently wrong with any of these goals or products, but when they become the intention of a yoga practice they destroy the heart of yoga. It is no longer about our union of our will with God's, but about furthering our own will via hedonism and consumerism.

To approach yoga with pure intention requires turning much of what society tells us about life and success on its head. A yogic state of mind not only recognizes the fallacy of competition in the "farther + faster = better" sense, but takes it a step further to the point that there is no place for competition in yoga. I was struck by the subtlety of this way of thinking once when a yoga teacher repeatedly issued the well-intentioned reminder, "Remember, in yoga the slowest one wins." I sat with that comment a moment, trying to pinpoint why it felt wrong. Then it hit me. She was simply manipulating the standard competition-based mindset of our culture to fit a yoga paradigm. There can be no winner/loser mentality in a yogic environment. It is very difficult for us to drop our habitual ways of thinking and being in the world.

I didn't begin my yoga practice with any awareness of the intention behind it. I just knew that I was drawn to it. And maybe that's enough when you're twenty-five. In retrospect, my intention and my motivation to practice were strongly rooted in a competitive attitude. I was naturally flexible, so with very little effort, I could "win" at the yoga game. Thankfully,

Sophia was moving me toward something bigger, but all I needed to know at that point was to keep coming back to the mat. I knew I felt better when I stepped off than when I stepped on.

Somewhere along the line, my personal faith began to solidify, and I began to make the connection between my yoga practice and my conscious contact with God. I had a faith family that was—blessedly—open to what I was learning. Soon I was teaching yoga classes in the gymnasium-turned-art-gallery in our church's reclaimed urban community center that had just months before been a crack house. I knew intuitively that doing yoga in this sacred space, surrounded by art and moving alongside those who shared my vision of faith, was what yoga was all about. Moments in which my faith is illuminated through the practice of yoga is what kept me coming back through pregnancies, colic, and all the chaos and joy that life with young children brings.

Regardless of your current life situation—a house full of children, a stressful job, or an empty nest—we all need a way to wholly focus ourselves—body, mind, and spirit—on God's will for our lives. Do you have to have yoga to do this? Of course not. Yoga is not an end in itself, only a vehicle we may use on our journey. Like many others, I have found a welcome peace in yoga's ability to nourish the spirit while calming the mind and strengthening the body. It's a powerful combination. Powerful even when practiced in its secular form, in a brightly lit yoga class at a fitness chain with an instructor who has never even heard of the ancient yogic sages.

Imagine taking that same hour and making it a sacred experience—using it to focus your attention on God's will for you. Giving yourself permission to just be in her presence, savoring the breath she's given you, calming your mind and stretching yourself beyond your previous physical limits. With an understanding of what yoga is, we can take its form and easily adapt it to a spiritual practice that can work within any religious framework—from Christianity to Buddhism, and beyond.

First, let's be clear—in spite of its current surge in popularity, yoga is not a trend or a fad. More people may be practicing it in the West now, but yoga would not vanish like the Jazzercise classes of the '80s and '90s (think striped leg warmers and sweatbands) if these new converts all rolled up their mats and stopped practicing today. Yoga is, in fact, an ancient system of postures, beliefs and practices which has been around since 3,000 BC. Like many con-templative spiritual practices dating back thousands of years—the Christian traditions of *lectio divina* and Benedictine psalmody, for instance—it works as well now as it did then. Unfortunately, many of the calming, centering, sacred practices of both Eastern and Western religions have been dismissed by our fast-paced, goal-oriented society.

Because yoga's roots are in the Hindu religion, many outside that realm have been, understandably, hesitant about trying it. In fact, many are out-right hostile toward yoga. I have all-too-frequently met people who con-sider yoga an occult practice and are genuinely afraid of it. The reality is that yoga is practiced by millions of people of many faiths all over the world. And while it did indeed originate, and initially flourish, in the cul-tural setting of India, yoga philosophy is not exclusively Hindu. Its spiritual application extend far beyond the purview of Hinduism.

In my own experience, I am drawn closer to God and am always more closely aligned with her vision for my life after a yoga class. I walk (or run) through the door, distracted and preoccupied. An hour and a half later, I am lying still, feeling my breath and thanking God for this moment. I am able to walk out of class and turn my will over to God much more easily than when I walked in because I have spent my class letting go and surren-dering, twisting and bending, listening to my inner voice, hearing Sophia speak. I have (temporarily) lost the need to be in control.

My goal is to dispel some of the fears and misconceptions about doing yoga as a Christian—or a person of any faith not historically linked to yoga via sutras, Vedas, mantras, and the other practices that bind Hinduism to yoga. Yoga slows down the wheels of the mind enough to for us to hear God speaking. Prayer is about talking to God. Yoga can put us in the right frame of mind to listen, regardless of which religion mediates the conversation.

You can, however, bring prayerful discernment to your yoga practice in an effort to live out your own faith authentically. You may encounter things that you will need to filter through your own belief system. But isn't that the way it always is in this world in which God's called us to live? Basically, hold tight to what sounds like God speaking to you and let go of all the rest. There are dozens of different schools of yoga and yogic phi-losophy, incorporating varying degrees of the Hindu-influenced culture in which it developed. Regardless of the type of yoga being taught, a teacher's perspective and belief system (and how much of that he or she brings into class) will affect your comfort level.

Also, be aware that your own internal barometer and personal preferences will change over time, evolving and fluctuating along with other facets of your practice. Traditional Sanskrit chants may agitate and distract you with their unknown meanings, while at other times you may find them extremely calming. Look at all your yoga teachers as guides who bring you something that you need. It may only be one small life lesson, but it is something you need to learn, process, or experience. You may take one class with that teacher or you may stick with that class and its teacher for decades. The introspective nature of yoga has a way of teaching us about ourselves, and in the process it, helps us discern what is true for us and what is not.

In Chapter 2, a bird's eye view of Patanjali's eight limbs of yoga, which form the basis of modern yogic philosophy, will help you become a discerning participant in your yoga practice. Once you understand the foundational precepts, you'll have the awareness you need to find the yoga resources that are right for you—whether it's a teacher, a class, a book or DVD.

In Chapter 3, we will take the traditional yoga model and place it in a contemplative context by looking at it in relation to historical Judeo-Christian practices: chanting, mantras, mysticism, and hesychasm—which have been all-but-lost in the world of modern Western religion. The application of this contemplative yogic paradigm will help create a yoga practice that will not compromise religious beliefs, but will enhance them by providing a safe haven for opening up, slowing down, and stretching beyond your limitations—physical, mental, and spiritual.

In his obscure doctoral thesis published in Bangalore in the 1990s—*Yoga Spirituality: A Christian Pastoral Understanding*—Cheirian Puthenpura manages to connect the heart of yoga to Christian spirituality in a way that compromises neither the ancient art of yoga nor the profound faith of the Christian believer. While the book's scope goes into very specific areas of interest to pastors tending their sick parishioners, the ground work he lays in bridging the gap between the worlds of Christianity and yogic philosophy helped me envision melding the two in my own life even more profoundly.

According to Puthenpura, yoga is "yoking, uniting, an art and wisdom of being, a skill in meditation, a process of transforming consciousness, a state of being which is light and unity." So I ask, as Christians, as Jews, as Buddhists and as Hindus, don't we want to be yoked to God? Wouldn't we love to be able to pray and meditate on God's words and will without being distracted by the stuff that clutters our daily lives? To maintain the transformed consciousness we feel in those moments that we truly connect with God? Don't we cherish those moments when we feel lightened from having entrusted our lives to God—having taken even just one of our fears, one of our seemingly insurmountable problems, and given it to God?

Matthew 11:30 says: "For my yoke is easy and my burden is light." When the worries of the world wash over me, I know I can do yoga, I can surrender that hour, re-yoke myself to God's will and emerge from that hour feeling lighter. Thanks be to God.

The Veda Sanskrit glossary defines yoga as "the joining of the *atma*, our individual soul, with the *paramatma*, the soul with God." Looking at the traditional eight limbs of yoga, we find the underlying philosophy shows numerous means of joining with God. Only one involves the physical postures which have come to embody in the West.

Yoga is a comprehensive philosophical system. In general, we get a very watered down version of it here in the United States. We know yoga as a system of postures, maybe complemented by some breathing exercises. The practice of yoga in India and other Eastern regions, which began three centuries before Christ was born, is so much more. The *asanas* (yoga postures) are only one of the eight limbs that make-up the traditional system of yoga as documented by Patanjali in the first—and still most revered—guide to the practice of yoga in 200 AD. These eight limbs include:

1. Yama: Universal morality
2. Niyama: Personal observances
3. Asanas: Body postures
4. Pranayama: Breathing exercises, and control of prana
5. Pratyahara: Control of the senses
6. Dharana: Concentration and cultivating inner perceptual awareness
7. Dhyana: Devotion, Meditation on the Divine
8. Samadhi: Union with the Divine

YAMA (THE FIVE "ABSTENTIONS"—ALSO REFERRED TO AS UNIVERSAL MORALITY): NON-VIOLENCE, NON-LYING, NON-COVETOUSNESS, NON-SENSUALITY, AND NON-POSSESSIVENESS

Grasping *yama* is a simple leap for anyone from a Judeo-Christian back-ground. These are the "don'ts" of ethical behavior. Translated literally, *yama* means "death"—in this case, the death of undesirable behaviors and traits. We're used to adhering (or at least trying our best to adhere to) a set of rules that tells us what not to do. The *yama*, combined with the next branch (*niyama*: the "dos"), are reminiscent of the ten commandments of the Judeo-Christian faith traditions and can be found almost verbatim on Moses' stone tablets. A close examination reveals these similarities:

Yama of non-violence (*ahimsa*): This would be analogous to the com-mandment, "You shall not kill." Even with this seemingly irrefutable, moral-ly universal admonishment, there are endless applications of this principle in the real lives of people around us.

One person may find squashing a bug reprehensible, while another may brandish a fly swatter with no compunction. Some people choose not to eat meat and consider violence against animals to be included in that commandment. Others are happy sitting down to a big, thick juicy steak and don't consider that an infringement of the commandment. Some go as far as to shun leather products, while others aren't bothered at that level. There are women who have had abortions and are at peace with their decision. There are also those who have had them and are not at peace, feeling that they personally violated their own standard of non-violence. There are those who advocate for euthanasia arguing that it can sometimes be the most humane choice; while others argue that it is never a humane choice. There are parents who teach kids not to hit by spanking them; and then there are those who see that as a blatant contradiction and an infliction of violence.

As much as we'd sometimes like to play God and have all the answers for everyone, the only answers we will ever really have are our own—and even that takes a tremendous amount of work, vulnerability, and an uncomfortable level of self-honesty. The important thing to remem-ber, as we move through the *yama* and the *niyama* (or through the ten commandments), is that it is God's job to establish the rules by issuing the commandments—the *yama*, the *niyama*, or whatever you choose to call them. As in much of life, the terminology is less important than the intent or the core meaning. We are not charged with setting the rules, but merely with understanding them and incorporating them into our lives.

Yama of non-lying (*satya*): "You shall not bear false witness against your neighbor." In plain English, "Don't lie." Paul drove home this key point again in Colossians when he admonished, "Stop lying to one another. What you have done is put aside your old self with your past deeds and put on a new self, one that grows with knowledge as it is formed anew in the image of its Creator" (Colossians 3:9-10).

Paul's statement represents a broader interpretation than Exodus 20:16, from which the commandment is taken. I have found that the Bible's richest teachings cannot be gleaned by taking a strictly literal interpretation. The Year of Living Biblically, A.J. Jacobs' intriguing personal chronicle of one man's humble quest to follow each of the 715 commandments found in the Bible to a tee—shows what true literalism looks like.

In this instance, the literal interpretation of the ninth commandment requires telling the truth while on the witness stand. How many times do most of us find ourselves called to bear witness for or against our neighbor? God used this commandment to point us in the right direction—in this case, to lead us to the truth. Telling the truth... living the truth... being the truth. Truth is an integral part of who Jesus is in his oft-quoted proclamation, "I am the way and the truth and the life" (paraphrase of John 14:6).

Truth inhabits our lives with many gray areas—those little white lies that make life run more smoothly, the omissions that keep the peace and even the magical experiences we weave for our children with characters like Santa Claus, the Easter Bunny, and the Tooth Fairy. It is not the letter of the law, but its intention, that we are charged with living out. Would Jesus begrudge us Santa Claus? Probably not. A huge proponent of child-like innocence, Jesus said, "Let the little children alone—let them come to me. The kingdom of heaven belongs to such as these" (Matthew 19:14). He clearly loved the innate joy of children.

Yama of non-covetousness (asteya): The grand finale of the ten commandments, the imperative against covetousness, is another one that was believed to have roots in the legal realm. Some Jewish Talmudic interpretations claim kidnapping was the offense against which this commandment was originally written. The act of coveting was also considered a precursor to the crimes that are prohibited by the commandments "Don't commit adultery" and "Don't steal." Focusing on the criminal avoidance aspect of this commandment helped people avoid the heart of the message contained within it. In any case, the admonition, as detailed almost identically in both Exodus 20:17 and Deuteronomy 5:21, includes a broad range of covetous behavior to guard against, saying, "No desiring your neighbor's house. No desiring your neighbor's spouse, or worker—female or male—or ox, or donkey or anything that belongs to your neighbor!" (Exodus 20:17).

As detailed as the list seems to be, it is not meant to be all-encompassing, as our capacity for covetousness is seemingly limitless. Hence the phrase "or anything that belongs to your neighbor" tacked onto the end. Coveting your neighbor's rooster or pig is not any less wrong than coveting the explicitly mentioned ox or donkey. Similarly, while *The Inclusive Bible* cited here does say "spouse," every other translation alludes only to "wives," leaving the women with no clearly stated prohibition against lusting after the husband next door.

This *yama*—and this commandment—is more subtle than the previous two because it operates in the realm of the mind, not necessarily advancing into physical actions like those involved in lying and violence. We all know that it is much easier to control our outsides (our actions) than to truly address our insides (our thoughts, emotions, and feelings). This one is about truly being at peace with where God has placed us, not just acting like we are by avoiding certain behaviors, like violence and lying. Later we will see how yoga offers some practical help with this interior work.

Yama of sensual restraint (bramacharya): Unlike the other *yama*, this is not a commandment of absolute avoidance; rather, it is a call to pursue sensuality in balance and within divinely sanctioned scenarios. Its application is even more personal than the other *yama*. For example, a monk or priest practicing *bramacharya* would be doing so with the goal of complete celibacy. A married person would be aspiring to faithfulness within the marriage; while a single person may be striving to postpone sexual expression until marriage, or whatever scenario was acceptable within their belief system.

This same sense of restraint applies to other sensual pleasures that can seize control of our will and our appetites—literally and figuratively. Chocolate is particularly seductive to me, but I can choose how I succumb to the temptation. Savoring fine, single-origin chocolate, one bite at a time, is a lovely pleasure; Sitting down and gorging on left-over Halloween candy in one sitting is a completely different experience, devoid of the sacred nature of the former. One embodies restraint, gratitude, and joy in simple pleasures, while the other espouses the cultural norms of gluttony and instant gratification. *Brahmacharya* does not prohibit us from indulging (even in the Halloween stash), but it does bring an awareness to our choice of indulgence.

The Sanskrit word for this *yama*—*brahmacharya*—can be broken down to reveal a broader interpretation of the *yama* so often associated with self-imposed limitations on earthly pleasures. "*Brahma*" is used to refer to God, while "*char*" means walk, and "*ya*" denotes an active approach. In this light, the often maligned *yama* transforms into the simple command to "walk with God."

Yama of non-possessiveness (*aparigraha*): This final *yama*—along with the previous four: non-violence, non-lying, non-coveting and sensual restraint—becomes an incredibly universal commandment once you begin comparing the sacred texts of different religions. This *yama* cannot be possessed by any one faith tradition because it is shared by so many.

While not precisely aligned with a specific commandment in the Judeo-Christian traditions, detachment from the craving to possess and hold something for ourselves is inherent in the commandments to "Make no idols," "Do not steal," and "Do not covet." The ideal of non-possession is the bedrock of the Buddhist faith which is built upon the concept of non-attachment as a core spiritual practice.

Christians tend to grasp our similarities with the Jews more easily than we do with those of other Eastern faiths—probably because we share the same sacred text. Our Old Testament is a close facsimile of the Hebrew Bible.

It is more difficult for many Christians to see how our faith is intertwined with other religions. We can get over-focused on distinctions that make "us" different from "them." In the years following September 11, 2001, we Americans have been unduly concerned with the extremist faction of the Muslim faith, defining a whole religion by the actions of a few fundamentalists.

While the Torah is familiar to many Christians, the Qur'an seems as foreign as the vedic scriptures on which much of yoga's philosophy is based. But the Qur'an echoes the ten commandments with very little variation from our own sacred text. While they are not enumerated as with the Christian Bible and the Jewish Torah, they can be found within the Qur'an as indicated below:

1. "There is no other god besides God" (Qur'an 47:19).
2. "My Lord, make this a peaceful land, and protect me and my children from worshiping idols" (Qur'an 14:35).
3. "And make not Allah's (name) an excuse in your oaths against doing good, or acting rightly, or making peace between persons; for Allah is One Who heareth and knoweth all things" (Qur'an 2:224).
4. "O you who believe, when the Congregational Prayer (Salat Al-Jumu`ah) is announced on Friday, you shall hasten to the commemoration of GOD, and drop all business" (Qur'an 62:9).
5. "....and your parents shall be honored. As long as one or both of them live, you shall never (even) say to them, "Uff" (the slightest gesture of annoyance), nor shall you shout at them; you shall treat them amicably" (Qur'an 17:23).
6. "....anyone who murders any person who had not committed murder or horrendous crimes, it shall be as if he murdered all the people" (Qur'an 5:32).
7. "You shall not commit adultery; it is a gross sin, and an evil behavior" (Qur'an 17:32).
8. "They shall not steal" (Al-Mumtahanah 60:12). And "The thief, male or female, you shall mark their hands as a punishment for their

41

crime, and to serve as an example from God. God is Almighty, Most Wise" (Qur'an 5:38).

9. "Do not withhold any testimony by concealing what you had witnessed. Anyone who withholds a testimony is sinful at heart" (Qur'an 2:283).

10. "And do not covet what we bestowed upon any other people. Such are temporary ornaments of this life, whereby we put them to the test. What your Lord provides for you is far better, and everlasting" (Qur'an 20:131).

Seeing these points of convergence among religions can be extremely comforting. The similarities point to something bigger and more powerful than any one religion can encapsulate within its boundaries. These synchronicities—these moments where tongues that speak different languages and find their sacred words in different books are all singing the same song—remind me that God is so much more than even the most sacred of scriptures can put into words. God cannot be contained within a system devised by humans.

This is one of the truths we could experience if we all belonged to a club like the one Rayna Idliby, Suzanne Oliver, and Priscilla Warner chronicled in their book *The Faith Club: A Muslim, A Christian, A Jew—Three Women Search for Understanding.*

Dr. William F. Vendley, Secretary General for the World Conference of Religions for Peace, recommends the book, saying, "Three contemporary women...search together across the divides of prejudice and fear. Their honesty becomes a path to connection; their courage leads into the ranges of the heart opened by their own religions. Working together, they each arrive where alone they could not go."

He is not describing a high-level religious summit organized by an international coalition to promote interfaith relations. This is just three moms sitting down and getting honest about their faiths, their backgrounds, and their fears. These are women just like us. What if people across the country started forming their own faith clubs? What if we intentionally sought out those with different beliefs, forged relationships, and engaged in authentic dialog while traversing the terrain of our differences, with the goal of arriving in a space where we can co-exist?

I am reminded of a Sufi tale used by Joan Chittister in her book *Called to Question*. She relays the story of Sufi disciples who, at their spiritual master's death bed, mourned his imminent departure, pleading, "If you leave us, Master, how will we know what to do?" In the beautiful, mystical way of the Sufis, the master replied, "I am nothing but a finger pointing at the moon. Perhaps when I am gone, you will see the moon." When I gaze at the moon, I find great joy in the knowledge that so many others are soaking up that same beauty. This is the essence of the final *yama* of non-possessiveness.

NIYAMA (THE FIVE "OBSERVANCES"): PURITY, CONTENTMENT, AUSTERITY, STUDY, AND SURRENDER TO GOD

While the *yama* tell us what to avoid, the *niyama* are designed to tell us which spiritual observances to pursue. We need both. A spirituality that gives rules without illuminating the path that draws us closer to God is an empty vessel. The *niyama* undertake this sacred task with a beautiful congruity to other sacred traditions.

Bible Gateway's commentary on Ephesians 4:25-28 captures this key concept perfectly saying, "Sinful desires and deceitful lust... promise men [and women] happiness, but render them more miserable and bring them to destruction if not subdued and mortified. These therefore must be put off, as an old garment, a filthy garment. They must be subdued and mortified. But it is not enough to shake off corrupt principles; we must have gracious ones." The *niyama*, as found in the Vedas and as lived out in Christ's life, are the gracious principles we must espouse to live a truly spiritual life.

The Inclusive Bible's translation of those same verses details several specific scenarios, illustrating the difference between ceasing to do bad and becoming a catalyst for good. In reference to theft, verse 28 admonishes, "You who have been stealing, stop stealing. Go to work. Do something useful with your hands, so you can have something to share with the needy." There is progression from delinquency to philanthropy. God wants us to live a life of extravagant grace—both given and received.

Niyamic guidance exists within the Judeo-Christian tradition, in the

commandments in which God sets forth specific spiritual observances—
"Honor your parents" and "Observe the Sabbath"—rather than issuing
commandments which shape our behavior through prohibitions. On a
larger scale, much of the New Testament is a living *niyama* communicated through Jesus' life. As we will see, every one of the *niyama*—purity,
contentment, austerity, study, and surrender to God—is found within the
character of Jesus Christ.

Niyama of Purity (*shaucha*)

Psalms 24:3-4 provides a vivid example of God calling us to purity:

> Who has the right to ascend YHWH's mountain?
> Who is allowed to enter YHWH's holy place?
> Those whose hands are clean
> and whose hearts are pure.

But what is this pure-heartedness to which God calls us? How do we
take it out of the book and put it into our lives? As is often the case, we
can get the answer by simply flipping ahead a few chapters and reading
about Jesus putting the concept into action.

Purity in Jesus' life is not to be confused with the cultural idea of es-
chewing all the temptations of the world. Jesus tells us to look inward for
the source and symptoms of our impurity. In Mark 7:15 Jesus says, "Nothing
that enters us from the outside makes us impure; it is what comes out of
us that makes us impure." He suggests we shouldn't worry so much about
being corrupted by the world. Instead, we should look at our thoughts,
attitudes, and behaviors to see if the purity we seek is there or not. If it is
there, it will be evident. If it is not, it will also be evident.

During Jesus' lifetime and the period leading up to it, adherence to
specific rules and guidelines qualified one as pure or impure. This was not
the evidence that Jesus considered when evaluating purity. As Jerome
Neyrey points out in his analysis of purity in Mark's gospel, "Jesus appears
to be out of place most of the time, dealing with people he should avoid,
doing unconventional things and not observing customs about places
and times." What mattered to Jesus was the purity of the thought and

underlying attitude that drove the behavior, not the behavior itself. In one well-known incident, Jesus showed that it was better to risk being considered impure by healing on the Sabbath than to leave someone hurting in order to adhere to the letter of the law (Mark 3:1-6).

The examples from Jesus' life leave us free to operate with grace in the world around us. In Jesus we find a role model who is unafraid of being contaminated by all that needs healing in this world. We find someone who walks into the areas that we are tempted to run away from. This way of living is equally applicable to our internal and external lives. Yes, Jesus wants us to go and do, to help and save, to give and serve; but he also wants us to enter those dark places in our own lives, to see what needs healing in our own hearts. These are two aspects of the same concept that Jesus taught through his life and his words.

To put it in yogic terminology, the public outreach, the healing of others, is the *yang*, while the inner seeking, the soul work, is the *yin*. The beauty of the *yin-yang* concept lies in the absolute intertwining of the two. One is not meant to exist without the other. This interdependence is a difficult concept to grasp and live out in a world so infused with *yang* and devoid of *yin*. James 2:20 speaks of faith without deeds being useless. Of course, the reverse is also true—deeds born out of impure motive, not rooted in fertile soil of faith, are equally useless. *The Message* translation of James 2:19-20 provide some vivid imagery for this concept:

> Do I hear you professing to believe in the one and only God, but then observe you complacently sitting back as if you had done something wonderful? That's just great. Demons do that, but what good does it do them? Use your heads! Do you suppose for a minute that you can cut faith and works in two and not end up with a corpse on your hands?

These powerful images communicate to us the extent to which the impure motives underlying a life of hypocrisy are absolutely incompatible with a spiritually healthy existence. As is the case with much spiritual grappling, the key is finding the balance between the motives (the *yin*) and the action (the *yang*).

Purity is to be lived, not earned or achieved. In the Christian faith, we often associate our symbolic baptismal rituals with the achievement of purity. It is important to remember that just as religion itself is not truth, but a system meant to point us to the truth, our rituals and our symbols are also signposts, not destinations. Baptism signifies our commitment to living with pure intentions, not a celebration of having reached a state of perpetual purity, or even a desire to do so. God provides us with another clue as to the connection between the birth of the divine and a state of purity with the choice of a virgin as the pure vessel through which Jesus is birthed. Indeed, our divine selves, the very best we are capable of, always surfaces when we are able to act with the purest of motives, becoming mere vessels through which God's plans can unfold.

Niyama of Contentment (*santosha*)

"The better part of happiness is to wish to be what you are." – Desiderius Erasmus (1466-1536)

When Jesus said, "He who comes to Me shall not hunger, and he who believes in Me shall never thirst," he was not talking about food and water. He was addressing the emptiness—the want and discontentment—that we have in our hearts. God designed human beings to be satisfied.

It is no coincidence that God delivers the same sense of divinely sourced contentment through Christianity as through other religions. Consider the *niyama* of contentment, the healing balm of the Psalms, the gentle reminder each time the word "Shalom" passes over Jewish lips on its way to a friend's ear, and the Muslim belief that the heart is the center of all God-consciousness and, therefore, of contentment. Listen closely and hear the multi-lingual voice of God speaking to all the inhabitants of the world in these ways and others.

God speaks contentment whether invited, acknowledged, embraced or ignored. Blessedly, God's behavior, character and message are not dependent upon our human perceptions or reactions. God speaks when we call out to Our Father, Our Mother, Our Savior or Our Breath of Life and just about any other moniker we could come up with.

Non-theistic religions like Buddhism are just as strongly rooted in contentment as a spiritual principle. The Buddha addresses contentment

46

directly in his Second Noble Truth, concluding that wanting deprives us of contentment and happiness. How closely his words resonate with Paul's in Philippians 4:10-12, "...for whatever the situation I find myself in, I have learned to be self-sufficient. I know what it is to be brought low, and I know what it is to have plenty. I have learned the secret: whether on a full stomach or an empty one, in poverty or plenty, I can do all things through the One who gives me strength."

The practice of yoga brings a physicality to the cultivation of contentment that is missing in almost all religious traditions. We seek contentment in our hearts through spiritual exercises, while our bodies—and often our minds—are working in opposition to our goal. Our culture shouts, "More, more, more!" while our hearts are yearning for a slower pace, whispering, "Enough...enough...enough." In his yoga sutras, Patanjali provides us with "movement or positions, breathing practices, and concentration, as well as the *yama* and *niyama*, [that] can contribute to a physical state of contentment (*santosha*)."

A 16th century sacred Sikh text reads, "Make contentment your earrings, humility your begging bowl, and meditation the ashes you apply to your body." What would life be like if we could put on an aura of contentment each morning as simply as clipping on a pair of earrings?

Niyama of Austerity (*tapas*)

"To have freedom is only to have that which is absolutely necessary to enable us to be what we ought to be." – Ibn Rahel (Medieval Christian chronicler)

The term austerity rolls awkwardly off our Western tongues, as if we are using a foreign language to recount memories of our Desert Mothers and Fathers whose relinquishment of worldly pleasures is unfathomable to our comfortable modern sensibilities. We look at religious ascetics' pursuit of eternal sanctity and see within their monastic walls a deprivation unrelated to our own lives.

It is not surprising then that we look outside the modern Westernized worldview for help in grappling with this elusive and misconstrued concept. The words here, attributed to Ibn Rahel, an Egyptian chronicler of Christianity who lived in the Middle Ages, point us in the right direction.

The statement doesn't say "To have freedom is to have *only* that which is absolutely necessary to enable us to be what we ought to be." It says, "To have freedom is *only* to have that which is absolutely necessary to enable us to be what we ought to be." Our black and white thinking wants to hear austerity and think, "must divest of worldly belongings." Once we realize we're not ready to do that, we dismiss the entire concept. The important thing is not that we shun everything peripheral to life, but that we hold tight to our core and keep ourselves centered within it.

The version with the misplaced "only" has a heavy, restrictive feeling, while the true quote has an expansive, light and optimistic tone to it. It sounds not only like something we could do, but like something to which we'd like to aspire. I am struck by the power of a simple word, properly placed, to transform us. Translation, too, can powerfully impact the interpretation of this *niyama*. Though typically translated as "austerity," the Sanskrit word "*tapas*" can also be mean "zeal" or "self-discipline." Christian yogini Bernadette Latin says:

> *Tapas* means that which generates heat. It is the practice of applying our energy and zeal toward the goal of union with God. Austerity and self-discipline may sound grim, but *tapas,* in the yogic tradition, is joyful positive action because it leads one to God. It is not self-punishment. It is self-control; it is the fiery determination each day to recommit one's self to the spiritual path and to the practices that foster spiritual growth.

When we consider this broader interpretation, we can see this *niyama* inviting us to include a modicum of self control in areas extending far beyond the realm of finance and consumption, with the ultimate goal being to free ourselves to focus on God's will for us.

So, how do we, as modern day Americans, relate to the concept of austerity? Mason Cooley provided this analogy: "Austerity causes constipation; excess, diarrhea." It's all about balance, a difficult position to obtain, both as individuals and as a culture. Austerity, in and of itself, is not an ideal, it's an extreme. Indeed, neither constipation nor diarrhea is ideal. Somewhere between the two is the healthy goal.

The movement toward simplicity in this country is growing. It's begin-ning to infiltrate every aspect of our lives, from spending to eating to housing and recreation. With fascination, I've followed folks who have em-barked upon personal quests to live without spending any money except for specified amounts designated for housing and food. They undertake this for a week, a month or even a year, and this is not an isolated or ex-tremist trend. Robert Passikoff predicted an end to the last bastion of ex-cess—deep discount splurges—saying, "Excessive spending, even on sale items, will continue to be replaced by a reason-to-buy at all." Awareness is starting to seep into our buying patterns, and awareness is a wonderful starting point for change.

Recent real estate headlines capture the move away from excess in the housing market: "New Homes Getting Smaller," "Say Goodbye to McMansions," and "Americans Buying Right-Sized Homes." I am particu-larly intrigued by the last one because it doesn't use the term down-siz-ing, which carries a connotation of deprivation. "Right-sizing" infers that homes are getting back in line with what we need, rather than providing all that is possible.

The experimentation with the principles of austerity extends to the table where gaps in our food chain are closing as we grow our own food, buy local and go organic. Hobby farms and urban edible gardens are be-coming more commonplace, and organic produce is making its way into mainstream grocery stores.

Just as we've found common ground with Jesus' teachings in each *yama* and *niyama*, so it is with austerity. In his Sermon on the Mount, Jesus tells followers, "Don't store up for earthly treasures for yourself, which moths and rust destroy and thieves can break in and steal. But store up for your-selves treasures in heaven, where neither moth nor rust can destroy them and thieves cannot break in and steal them. For where your treasure is, there will your heart be as well. ...No one can serve two superiors. You will either hate the one and love the other, or be attentive to one and despise the other. You cannot give yourself to God and Money" (Matthew 6:19).

Austerity, it seems, is both biblically and culturally relevant. Far from be-ing a relic from the past or a fringe practice, it is a breeze blowing through our lives brushing gently against us every time we say no to another pair of shoes that we don't need. Every time we decline that "free" line of credit. Or eat leftovers instead of going out to eat. It is mindfulness applied to our finances, but more importantly to our needs and our wants. Here's to learning the difference.

Niyama of Study (svadhyaya)

Esteemed yoga teacher Donna Farhi, in her book *Yoga Mind, Body & Spirit,* says that "any activity that cultivates self-reflective consciousness can be considered *svadhyaya* (Sanskrit for study)." In modern Christian lexicon this might be a Bible study. In the church's contemplative tradition, it could be a more sublime and experiential activity—walking a labyrinth, creating a personal enneagram, or participating in a *lectio divina*. These contemplative options for incorporating study into our spiritual lives embody a wholeness that's missing from the intellectual path forged by many within Western religious life. Study within mainstream religion consists primarily of listening to speakers, reading books, and talking about it all. Making space for that new knowledge to take root in our lives leads us into *svadhyaya*.

Growing up in a traditional Christian environment, I wasn't introduced to the type of spiritual practices that would have led me to *svadhyaya*. I found certainties where I longed for mystery. I was given answers that didn't fit and had questions that weren't permitted. All was not well with my soul. It was on my yoga mat that I first encountered the mystical side of God and began carving out spaces where God's voice could echo freely through my whole being.

I discovered that head knowledge only penetrates so deeply and often wriggles out of my grasp just as easily as it flowed into my mind. Cultivating practices that help us hang onto all the book smarts is the spiritual equivalent of Waldorf education, a century-old, deceptively simple educational philosophy which works purposefully in the realms of the head, heart, and hands—engaging the intellect, spirit, and dexterity, while acknowledging that wisdom gained through only one of these will quickly fade. In an educational setting, this may be accomplished as children create delicate water color paintings or rhythmically knit while a beloved fable is being told (not read) in an engaging and animated fashion. Take a moment to think about what a fully engaged spirituality would look like in your life.

To fully grasp this *niyama*, I had to leave behind the belief that to study meant to seek external knowledge and claim it for our own. Limiting the search for truth to outside sources—books, the Internet, sermons, lectures, others' opinions—can be dangerous territory. The most important study we can ever do is internal. It is also precisely the work that we often try to avoid. It is so much easier to absorb from the environment than to explore the landscape of the soul.

My yoga teacher tells the tale of a precocious four-year-old who announced to his mom, "You're not the boss of me!" No one—not our teacher, pastor, priest or rabbi—is the boss of us. They're not our Higher Power or our God, and if we try to make them into these things, we are certain to be disappointed. No one—absolutely no one—can tell anyone else the inner truths about herself. Close friends can speak their truths into our lives, sending rays of light ricocheting off the walls of the soul, illuminating things a bit. A gifted preacher or speaker, similarly, can point us in the right direction, crafting familiar stories into new creations that open our eyes to truths that were already hiding somewhere deep within.

So when I just wanted my teacher to tell me the right way to do the pose—because I was upside down, backwards and unable to figure it out for myself—she refused, saying with a smile, "I'm not the boss of you." She knows me well enough to know that I don't *really* want someone telling me what to do and how to do it. So, instead, she gently placed my hand on my back and asked me to feel my alignment and make my own adjustment. Directional touch, she called it. To me, it was the *niyama* of study in action.

This internal work is not a foreign concept and is compatible with Jesus' teachings and Jewish midrashic writings. Like the other limbs of yoga, the idea behind this *niyama* flows from and through Christian tradition. John Calvin proclaimed in his Institutes for Christian Religion, "Nearly all the wisdom we possess, that is to say, true and sound wisdom, consists of two parts: the knowledge of God and of ourselves."

Perhaps one reason this teaching often seems lost to those of us in contemporary Christian churches is because the best teachings on the idea that knowing ourselves and knowing God are inexorably intertwined are found in the so called "lost" gospels. Most prominently, they can be seen in the Gospel of Thomas, the compilation of sayings attributed to Jesus that begins: "Jesus said if you seek the Kingdom of God in the sky then the birds will precede you. And if you seek it in the sea, then the fish will precede you, but the Kingdom is in you. And if you know yourself then you know the Kingdom of God. But if you don't know yourself, you live in poverty."

This scriptural exaltation of self-study as absolutely necessary to spiritual growth is the *svadhyaya* fuel that we find in the mystical traditions of all religions. The Gospel of Thomas and other contemplative texts point us inward, taking our focus off the external sources of wisdom and leading us into our souls, where Sophia is waiting.

Niyama of Surrender to God (*ishvarapranidhana*)

This culmination of the *niyama* echoes Jesus' supreme commandment to "Love the Lord your God with all your heart and with all your soul and with all your strength and with all your mind; and love your neighbor as yourself" (Luke 10:27). Its position as the final *niyama* is not accidental. In fact, all the previous *yama* and *niyama* equip us with the tools to carry it out. Contrary to its passive-sounding admonition, surrendering to God is an act that requires an understanding and adherence to all the other *niyama* to be successful.

We begin with abstaining from abhorrent behavior by practicing the *yama* of non-violence, non-lying, non-covetousness, non-sensuality, and non-possessiveness. Then we embrace the *niyama* of purity, contentment, austerity and study. All of this leads us to a the climactic final *niyama* of surrender to God.

The form of Christianity I grew up with positioned surrender as a one-time deal played out in the blazing moment of glory when we accepted Jesus into our hearts and were propelled forward to the front of the church. Conversion-driven evangelism tells us that once we have surrendered, we're "in" and can check that box off. When I didn't feel fully surrendered after I became a Christian at age eleven, I just took another walk down the aisle in college and found myself in the baptismal being washed clean—again.

Now I understand surrender not as a moment but as a way of life. It must be done again and again—sometimes many times in a day... or even in an hour. And it doesn't just happen in baptismal waters. It happens every time we choose to set aside our own agenda, our petulant self-will—our best-laid plans—and turn life over to a God we trust even more than our own schemes and plots. In surrendering we acknowledge that we are not the authors of our own lives, merely the actors on the stage. We are either going off our own script or following God's. The irony is that when we follow God's script, we become who we were truly meant to be rather than an ego-driven shadow of our divinely inspired selves. This encapsulates the beauty of surrendering to God.

Because I have a faith in a God that is bigger than my thoughts, I can ask for help in dealing with them, even when they carry me to unruly spots. Sophia may rush in and whisk the offending thoughts away. Then again, she might cause them to linger, sending me an important message. She might use them to turn on a light bulb in my head, illuminating an answer that had been eluding me. The point is that I have to surrender to God for any of this to happen. If I don't, I'm still relying on my own imperfect intellect or intuition to banish or hold tight to thoughts that visit me. Again, we see that this *niyama* is not at odds with Christianity's aim, but in harmony with its admonition to surrender to God.

Christianity is supremely adept at redeeming life's inevitable suffering without trying to eradicate it from our lives. We have Jesus as the example that guides us through those spots where we feel as if we've been abandoned and left hanging. Those are the moments where surrender seems an impossible feat but is the one action we can take that will make a real difference in our lives.

Surrender is easy when everything is going our way. It is an overlooked miracle lost in the chaos when things are falling apart.

Again, falling back on the lyrical genius of singer/songwriter Carolyn Arends, I find this affinity we have with Jesus' suffering in her words, "There's a Man of Sorrows, acquainted with our grief. And he's done his share of crying in the night with no relief. There isn't any heartache that he has not known." While I may never grasp why God's plan had to include Jesus' crucifixion, these lyrics remind me that there is no grief too deep for Jesus. I can see his suffering redeemed every time someone sees their own pain mirrored on his face and reflected back in a pool of divine light. That light makes it safe to surrender.

ASANA: LITERALLY MEANS "SEAT," AND IN PATANJALI'S SUTRAS REFERS TO THE SEATED POSITION USED FOR MEDITATION

Most Westerners begin and end their yoga practice at this third limb. Looking at yoga in a holistic way, it seems incongruous that this third limb should be singled out as the essence of the practice and termed "yoga" in and of itself. In fact, when looking at it in context, *asana* is actually a pre-paratory stage of a yoga practice, designed to ready a practitioner for the breathing and meditation to follow. After examining the *yama* and the *niyama* that serve as the foundation for a yoga practice, it seems almost irreverent to disregard them and rush to the poses. The tendency in the West to take this short cut is indicative of our goal-oriented mentality: to get to the pay off with as little work as possible—especially the messy work of spirituality. Our very *yang* performance-driven psyches may pro-pel us to the mat for power yoga, while all-too-often our soul just wants the *yin* experience of sitting and meditating.

The term *asana* in fact, when traced back to Patanjali's sutras origi-nating in approximately 200 BCE, refers specifically to the seated posi-tion designed for meditation. Practicing this particular *asana* repeatedly was done to allow the practitioner to extend the time they could spend seated in meditation. *Asanas* have expanded exponentially over the past 2,000 years. Today you are just as likely to find a yoga practitioner stand-ing, lying, or upside down as you are to find them seated.

Still, Patanjali's imperative holds true. *Asanas*, by nature, are meant to be firm, but relaxed. A challenging paradox to our Westernized minds. Regardless of the position assumed it should not be painful. If we go into a pose that causes us pain, we are violating the very first *yama* of *ahimsa*, or non-violence.

A yoga practice takes on a whole new dimension when the *yama* and *niyama* are studied and applied to the *asanas*. The *asanas* can then be-come less like physical exercise and more like life lessons. We can con-template how to look for the truth in our poses, rather than trying to make them look right (*satya*). We can work on not coveting that perfectly executed pose on the mat next to us (*asteya*). We can take the focus off of the desires that show up, even on our mats, in the form of rumbling stomachs or overactive libidos (*bramacharya*). We can maintain a posture of non-possessiveness or exclusivity as we devote our practice to God, remembering that we don't own the concept or understand it any better than those with different faith systems (*aparigraha*).

The *niyama* follow seamlessly with the intention of practice naturally becoming more pure (*shaucha*) as the *yama* are applied. We can become content (*santosha*) in our practice because we are no longer coveting what is not ours. We know we already have what we need (*tapas*), and we are open to the lessons that will penetrate deeply (*svadhyaya*) as we surrender to God (*ishvarapranidhana*).

Simply by approaching practice in that way, we can embody the yogic philosophy which may have previously seemed bafflingly exotic, beyond our reach, or out of our comfort zone. Just by bringing the *yama* and *niyama* onto the mat with us, we are primed to become students of life who use their yoga mats as a classroom, not a workout room.

So, why so many different poses? If the one seated position was good enough for yoga's Patanjali and his fellow practitioners, why not just sit around, breathing and chanting? Well, in a nutshell, life was simpler then. More active yoga has taken hold in the West because it harnesses our abundance of *yang* energy, gently guiding it, stretching it (and us), while leading us to a place where, finally, at the end of class, we are able to lie down in *savasana* (corpse pose) and give ourselves permission to just be there in stillness for a few minutes. This is not a treat we earn for having made it through the more rigorous poses. It is, indeed, the point of those rigorous poses.

America is a smorgasbord of opportunities, cultures and people, and its approach to yoga reflects that. A seemingly infinite variety of yoga classes exist here—Iyengar, Forrest, Power, Vinyasa, Yin, Restorative, Bikram and more. This can be overwhelming, but we can be thankful for the options and explore them joyously. There is something to be gleaned from almost every approach to yoga. Your personal needs and temperament at any given point in your life will make different schools appropriate at different times. Build up a repertoire by trying many different styles, and you will have a yoga toolkit from which to draw when you need it.

Restorative at the end of a tough week. Vinyasa to get your juices flowing. Yin when you need to cultivate your more introspective qualities. Power yoga when you need to burn off some steam or summon some yang energy. Iyengar when you want intentionality and precision to bring balance to a chaotic life. If you're craving some intensity pop into a Forrest class that will push you to your limits.

This chart summarizes several major yoga styles, including the spiritual fruit most directly correlated with each one. Naturally, real life yoga is not as black and white as this, and the spiritual fruits overlap and appear in each form of yoga at different times for different practitioners. Each of these styles is a sub-set of the over-arching label of *hatha* yoga, which denotes a practice focused on the physical body.

YOGA STYLE	DESCRIPTION	SPIRITUAL FRUIT
Vinyasa	breath and asanas are connected, almost orchestrally, in flowing sequences	grace
Power	vigorous, fitness-based vinyasa practice designed to meld with Western desire to bring yoga to gyms (traditionally called Ashtanga yoga)	commitment
Iyengar	precise focus on body alignment with the aid of props and the integration of the eight limbs of yoga	release of ego
Forrest	an intense approach, including long holds and extended standing series, emphasizes connecting to feelings in order to work through physical and emotional trauma	inspiration
Yin	mostly sitting or lying postures for promoting growth, clearing energetic blockages, and enhancing circulation	serenity
Restorative	the body is supported, using props, to provide a deep sense of relaxation in extended supine poses	self-love

My one caveat in endorsing all types of yoga would be to look at the intention behind the system and to how that's translated by the teacher. You can rely on your intuition to guide you on this. If a class feels ego-driven or unhealthy for you, listen to that. A good litmus test of a class is to see if the *yama* and *niyama* are upheld. Are you being asked to push beyond your own healthy limits? Does the yoga being taught allow for self-study or does it impose its own agenda? Does the school of yoga or the founder's personality seem to supersede the personal practice? A "yes" to any of these questions might make you reconsider the class or teacher you've chosen.

There are exercise systems that pluck yoga postures and combine them with some other form of non-spiritual exercise—yoga-lates (yoga and pilates) and yollet (yoga and ballet), for example. These are very legitimate ways of sculpting and shaping your body, but they should not be confused with yoga practices. I find myself agitated when I'm traveling and track down a yoga class only to find myself doing "yoga crunches" or calisthenic leg lifts between my up and down dogs. When talk turns to toning and firming as an intention, the spiritual part of the practice has been lost.

Asanas are, by definition, the most physical manifestation of a yoga practice. But all the physicality should be focused on the larger intention of alignment which—when we recognize that the mind, body and spirit are inseparable—has far-reaching implications that go way beyond six-pack abs or a firm tush. Physical alignment is simply a tangible way for us to work toward aligning the more subtle areas of our selves. *Asanas* become tools that we can use to access those hard-to-reach places. The dark spots we don't like to to visit or even acknowledge.

This is exactly where Sophia emerges from the shadows, the embodiment of divine wisdom wrapped in serenity. Living yoga—all eight limbs—provides both a way and a space for facing deeply buried fears and unacknowledged heartaches with the assurance that all will be well.

Thoughts of our body in yoga always linger around the spots where discomfort arises and we sense misalignment. Perhaps the cause of the misalignment is in our intention which is ego-infused and pushing us too far. Remembering the *yama* of non-violence, *ahimsa*, we back off.

Perhaps the discomfort stems from within our physical body, and we

57

need to pull our muscles in closer to the bones, lengthen our spine or plant our feet more firmly. All these actions cause us to be aware of where we are at that moment—and to be truthful about it, practicing the *yama* of truth (*satya*) in our body and in relation to the space around us. Rather than projecting us into some imagined state of future fitness (with visions of our bikini-clad selves strolling a beach), they keep us firmly grounded in the present.

PRANAYAMA: THIS KEY CONCEPT IN YOGA TEACHES US TO GET IN TOUCH WITH OUR PRANA (VITAL ENERGY OR LIFE FORCE) THROUGH THE PRACTICAL WORK OF THE BREATH

The fourth limb, *pranayama,* together with the *asanas* constitutes the basis for virtually every type of yoga class you will encounter in the West. Few venture beyond these two limbs, though some will include a bit of the seventh limb, *dhyana,* or meditation.

This realm then becomes the heart of *hatha* yoga for practitioners in our part of the world. In the context of the larger yogic philosophy, these branches are powerful *yang* aspects. We may not think about gentle yoga poses, breathing, and meditating as *yang*, but when we look at them next to the subtler, more philosophical limbs of the *yama, niyama,* and other devotional practices, they are the more action-oriented limbs. *Asana, pranayama,* and meditation all have a prescriptive nature and a defined space—a yoga mat or *zafu* (meditation pillow)—upon which to carry them out. They lend themselves to class formats and lay the groundwork for the integration of balancing *yin* aspects of spirituality—whether that spirituality comes from a yoga practice, faith tradition or both.

Practically speaking, we use the breath in yoga to follow the flow of energy through our body. To observe it first, and then to try to redirect it, experimenting and playing with the energy we embody. Like its external counterpart, the wind, breath is most easily observed by the tale tell signs it leaves as it passes. Picture the wind rustling the leaves on a tree, giving us goosebumps as it ushers us from summer warmth to winter chill.

Likewise, our breath rushes into our nostrils in a cooling burst, bringing in fresh energy along with scents from the space within which we exist. Connecting us to those around us, our breath becomes a more intimate version of the winds that whip around the globe, giving no credence to man-made borders. We all share the same air, breathing it in and out in a communal, life-giving act. One to which we rarely give a thought.

When we undertake a *pranayama* practice, we give our breath the attention it deserves. Instead of mindlessly barreling through our day, we stop and notice the breaths that, strung together, make up our lives.

Because of the holistic nature of yoga, it is virtually impossible to separate the practice of yoga from the practice of *pranayama*. I have heard in more than one yoga class that your breath is your yoga. If you are not using your breath in your practice, you may be exercising, but you're not doing yoga. Yoga—true to its root meaning of "yoke"—uses breath to link us to the present moment and also to the divinity within us. Rather than intellectualizing the concept of God, that rational process is relinquished to the rhythm of the breath. Somehow, when I let go of trying to label and understand God, I finally come face-to-face with an amazing flow of energy. Sophia shows up, tethering me to the present.

Just taking a moment to notice the relief even one deep breath brings can alter the trajectory of your day. You can cultivate gratitude for that breath even if everything outside you seems to be falling apart. Instead of joining in the chorus announcing that the sky is falling, you can choose a different response, one based on the calmness you are experiencing inside rather than the chaos going on around you.

I always loved that fable about Chicken Little's histrionics brought about by a misinterpreted acorn. Like many of the lessons we hold dear, the story is found in other cultures. Buddhist scripture tells the story of a hare that starts a stampede among the animals when a wayward piece of fruit drops on his head. The hare, like Chicken Little, wrongly assumes that the world is coming to an end. How different the endings of both tales would have been if the hysterical protagonists would have stopped and taken a deep breath before reacting.

When you practice *pranayama* on your mat, you can be sure it will wind its way into the rest of your life in wonderful, unexpected ways. My favorite surprises in this realm come from my kids. I see them using *pranayama* as tools in their lives just when things get overwhelming—for them or for me—and it makes me smile. In lieu of the traditional time out chair set in some dark corner of the house, my daughter used to go out and sit by a tree in our yard to do the "bunny breathing" that I had taught her. As I watched her breathing in and out, her little nose wiggling, her tension seemed to melt away.

My son told me recently that he taught a spirited and active friend of his to stop and take a deep breath when impulsivity got the best of him during class. With a discreet hand signal that could be given from across the room, he would remind his friend to take a deep breath to regain control—a tool I've encouraged him to use over and over again himself.

Pranayama is a tool that any one of us—even our kids—can use just by stopping and remembering to use the breath we're all blessed with. We can experiment with *pranayama* in its more formal form with any number of breathing exercises that can be done before, during, or after an *asana* practice.

Common *pranayamic* terms and practices include:

Ujjayi **Breathing...** This is the intentional breath you use throughout your *asana* practice. With *ujjayi* breathing, you breathe in and out through the nose, never through the mouth. Because it comes from deep within, it reverberates gently through the body. When I first began studying yoga, I was told it should sound like Darth Vader. Now I know a less aggressive form—think purring kitten—is a healthier way to practice.

Modulated Breathing... Once you've established your *ujjayi* breath, you can experiment with the length of your inhales and exhales. Begin by breathing with equally matched in and out breaths. Then hold breath for equal counts between the two. A good starting point is four seconds for each segment—four seconds in, four seconds holding, and four seconds out. Eventually, you can work up to a more difficult pattern of a shorter inhale (two seconds) and longer exhale (four seconds). Finally, when you've mastered this, you can add a break of eight seconds during which you hold your breath between the inhale and exhale.

Alternate Nostril Breathing... You might be surprised to know that we all favor one nostril over the other. Every yoga practice works to

60

balance some part of our being. Alternate nostril breathing brings equilibrium to our breath, distributing it more evenly throughout our bodies. Beginners can start with five sets of this cleansing and balancing practice, which begins with *ujjayi* breathing in a comfortable seated position. The right palm is then turned up, the pointer and middle fingers curled toward the palm. This leaves the thumb, ring and pinky fingers to work with. Closing the left nostril with the ring, and pinky fingers, the practitioner breathes in slowly (two seconds) through the right nostril, then closes it with the thumb, releasing the ring and pinky finger from the left nostril, exhaling for a count of four. The pattern is then repeated on the other side.

Just as religion uses various tools—worship, scripture and prayer, among others—to point you to God, *pranayama* uses your breath to connect you with the energy flow in your body that might otherwise go undetected. You might discover a secret reservoir of joy ready to burst through to the surface, triggered by a new awareness or receptiveness. You may find an old hurt, buried and yearning to be released. Tears—of joy or sadness—may flow.

Pranayama is a means, not an end. Like God, our *prana* (or energy) is invisible and often silent (unless it gets our attention with illness or anxiety), but if we learn to tune in, it is possible to to uncover the secrets of our own spirit with the same wonder we find when religion reveals God to us in a new way. In fact, it is through this deep awareness that we begin to feel God at work in our being. We can enter into a new level of honesty with ourselves (*satya*, the yama of truthfulness) and stop disconnecting our physical form from its spiritual undercurrents. In essence, we can become whole again.

This is not to say that we will always like what we discover or that if we are tuned into our *prana* things will always flow smoothly and, our bodies will stay disease and pain-free. The disease and pain might hold a message for us that can only be communicated through the discomfort they bring. Indeed, it is in meeting these difficult situations with an equanimity bolstered by deep breaths that we are transformed.

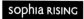

PRATYAHARA: THE PRACTICE OF TUNING INTO THE SENSES WITH CONTROL AND DISCERNMENT; WITHDRAWING, SO THAT WE MAY BE FULLY PRESENT TO THE REALITY IN WHICH WE FIND OURSELVES

As a child, I suffered from migraines which caused nausea that would go on for days. Instinctively, I developed a practice that I can recall vividly. I would lay—more often than not on the bathroom floor where I spent much time during those spells—and envision all the pain in my head collecting into a glowing red ball. I then used my mind to move the ball out of my body, holding it just above my head, where it floated. While I held it there—actively controlling the flow of energy in my body—I was blessedly free of pain. It took a lot of concentration, but the pay-off of a few minutes of pain relief was worth it.

Am I grateful for years of migraines? No, but I can see that they allowed me to access a part of my being that I would not have discovered otherwise. I can look back on almost all of the difficulties in my life and find something in each of them that brought new understanding of something.

Pratyahara is the withdrawal or subtle control of the sense organs. *Pranayama* prepares us and is a gateway leading us to *pratyahara*. While focusing on your breath, you are narrowing your sensory load by ignoring all the other stimulus around you. The myriad of stimuli around you are not disappearing, but through the direction of your attention, you are, effectively, eliminating them from your consciousness—at least for the moment.

That's exactly what I was doing when I consciously removed myself from my migraine pain as a child. There is no need to wait for a crisis situation to employ this powerful tool. Trying to dissipate the stress that had been building in me for a few days during the holidays, I walked out to the edge of a wooded area and listened, really listened. I closed my eyes and surrendered my sight. I didn't take note of the scents blowing toward me. I banished the to-do list that had been running through my head. The mocking voice saying, "You'll never get it all done!" vanished. I heard birds, unconcerned about Christmas cards or shopping lists, carrying on lively conversations. I imagined what they might be saying. I listened to the cold winter air rustling the grasses and trees. I heard larger animals—raccoons? rabbits?—moving through the underbrush, and squirrels scampering in the canopy above. The whole experience—a simple *pratyahara* practice—lasted less than five minutes, but it left me refreshed and ready to move through my day less frantically.

Pratyahara works just as well when applied to the other senses as it does to hearing, of course. One of my favorite applications is the Benedictine practice of mindful eating. If you want to home in on the experience of taste, try slowly and silently eating a bowl of soup on a cold night. Not only will you savor the taste of the soup as it moves over your tongue, but the warmth of it will move through your body, extending the experience beyond that of a meal where we eat and move on to another bite, another thought, another activity before the food is even down our throats.

While soup is soothing and a great way to ease into mindful eating, you can expand your experience into a seasonal rhythm. Soup is perfect for a winter practice. A salad full of the first greens of spring can usher in the warming winds of the season, awakening our taste buds to the delicate treats ahead. Juicy strawberries and peaches, dripping from our chins, call us to the informality of summer, while crunching into a crisp apple is the perfect way to transition our taste buds to back to the routine that fall brings with it. Who would have thought that yoga could be so delicious?!

We can create a beautiful weekly rhythm if we take one sense and focused on it each day. How much more will we appreciate the beauty we receive through each of them if we focus on one at a time? Monday could be our day to see the world. Tuesday we could listen to it. Wednesday we could taste it. Thursday breathe it in and savor its smell. And on Friday we could reach out and touch it, taking in its texture and its form.

We are inundated with an unprecedented amount of stimuli from more electronic devices than a previous generation could conceive. We have to constantly work to avoid sensory overload. If we follow the cultural norms, we're either going to be overwhelmed or anesthetized. And neither is a healthy option. By singling out one sense and allowing ourselves to focus on only the messages we are receiving via that sense, we can train ourselves to withdraw, and in doing so to appreciate what is around us with an intensity we couldn't muster otherwise.

Sensory experiences like relaxing baths, nature walks, and succulent food guide us toward the awareness we need to sit with ourselves. To be comfortable with what we will find should we dare to be quiet and listen.

In a purpose-driven culture, I am discovering it can be challenging to reach this level of awareness. Even in the spaces where we declare peace and calm should reign, chitter chatter invades.

I was at a spa recently, comfortably ensconced in my favorite spot, a candlelit room filled with chaise lounges and chenille throws. The Tranquility Room. There's even a sign on the door designating it as such. Despite the fact that it's explicitly set aside for quiet meditation, some people couldn't help themselves. Unable to rest in the peace of the room facilitated by the flickering flames in the fireplace and the trickling waters of the fountains flanking it, they stage whispered to each other. One woman checked her email and then read her emails out loud to a friend. Disconnection, even in a place set aside for such a state, was just not possible. It is a challenge for all of us.

Scores of people have confessed to me—with pride, frustration or a mixture of the two—that they can't meditate. They are just not the kind of person who can achieve that kind of stillness. There's not a gene that makes you the kind of person that is able to meditate or dooms you to a state of perpetual motion. Meditation is a practice we can choose to develop over time. And *pratyahara* is a very practical way to begin cultivating a meditative mind without having to sit in lotus or any other yoga posture. It's a living meditation that can transform the most ordinary aspects of your life into the most extraordinary moments you can imagine.

The first three limbs of yoga are the practical ones—the do's, the don'ts, and the physical movements. The fourth and fifth form the bridge that carries us from tangibility to deep spirituality, guiding us inward through our breath and our senses so that we might become living embodiments of Psalm 46:10, "Be still and know that I am God." The final three limbs can take us there in quiet contemplation, leaving us with a spirit-filled peace that is more personal, more intimate than any we've ever known.

To see a clear path through these final, highest branches, we have to look at the cultural and linguistic barriers that inhibit the divine intimacy we're seeking. Embedded within that simple psalm, "Be still and know that I am God," is a formidable barrier. We confuse knowing with knowledge. In a spiritual sense, they are very different concepts. We learn about God in Bible studies, Sunday school classes, and during weekly sermons. That is, we glean information about God's character, God's words, and God's deeds. This is knowledge *about* God. It is not knowing God.

The Western worldview is fixated on accumulating knowledge to facilitate material progress, and it downplays the importance of the deeper kind of spiritual knowing referenced in Psalm 46. And beyond the unique cultural construct of the American dream—brought to life in animatronic glory by Disney's classic Tomorrowland attraction, the Carousel of Progress—we are now part of a global economy where information, shared via the World Wide Web, is the currency. Having more information at our fingertips makes us more powerful in this reality, but doesn't have the same power in the spiritual realm.

So, how do we come to this spiritual knowing? As *pranayama* and *pratyahara* brought us to this place in our journey, the next limbs, *dharana* (concentration) and *dhyana* (meditation) will prepare us for *samadhi* (liberation), which will finally allow us to be still and know God. It is this deep, penetrating knowledge that is the wisdom of Sophia.

DHARANA (CONCENTRATION): FIXING THE ATTENTION ON A SINGLE OBJECT TO CULTIVATE INNER PERCEPTUAL AWARENESS

When I was a kid, I'd never heard of ADD. Today, estimates say that one out of ten kids is plagued with this phenomenon which leaves them in a perpetual state of distraction, leading to medication which leaves them anesthetized to the world with which they are trying to assimilate. If there was ever a point in history when we needed *dharana* practice, this is it.

In this more esoteric area of yoga, some people become cautious about the spiritual implications of the practice. *Dharana* is not about focusing on any object of religious significance. It is not about attuning yourself to an icon, idol, or other entity. It is merely, yet profoundly, the practice of choosing to anchor the energy of our mind to any practical focal point that you like; visual, tactile, auditory or olfactory.

My favorite—and earliest—experience with *dharana* is candle gazing. There is something intrinsically mesmerizing about a flickering flame. It is easy to be drawn into the dancing glow of a candle, forgetting the "to-dos" and the "what-ifs" that our minds return to if not focused. I try to end my day with this practice as often as possible, focusing on a salt crystal candle's undulating amber glow. I may only practice for a few minutes or I may challenge myself to more. As I expand this practice into longer stretches, I further hone my concentration. This is important because like a muscle, the ability to concentrate can weaken if we don't use it.

The more senses we are able to engage in this practice, the easier it is for us to keep ourselves anchored in the present. If our focal point provides something for all our senses to appreciate, there will be less room for distractibility. For example, an unscented candle will give you a visual focal point, but does not occupy the senses of smell, touch, taste, and hearing.

A scented candle, draws the sense of smell into the practice. And in front of a blazing fireplace or fire pit, you will not only see the flames, you will smell the smoke as it wafts toward you. You will feel the heat as it emanates, reaching for you. You will hear its crackling, and the wood settling as the fire burns on. The experience is elemental and organic—a perfect *dharana* experience.

The total integration of sensory experiences embodied by the fire is significant. I have experimented with visually focusing on one thing (my candle) while auditorily focusing on another (the steady trickling of my bath water draining from the tub). While both are calming when focused on individually, together they are distracting. The sound and the image aren't united, so the focus doesn't feel one-pointed either. Like watching a movie where the film and sound tracks don't match, it's distracting.

An organic, elemental subject is helpful in *dharana*. Focusing on something the comes from the earth, that was created by God, not by humans, brings a special kind of spirituality to the process. A space heater has many of the elements of a fire—heat and a warm glow. The fact that it vibrates with electricity instead of organic, life-giving energy, does not induce the same calming state conducive to meditation.

Melding two limbs, *dharana* can be cultivated on your mat during an *asana* practice by focusing on one very specific physical movement or alignment. For example, you may decide to focus on lifting your ribs as far away from your hips as you can in every pose you do during a class or home practice. You could stay attuned to this effort by keeping your attention on the space you are creating between each of your rib bones as they move up, creating length in your entire spine. You may not have the multi-sensory anchor that you can create in seated meditation, but the movement becomes your anchor, tethering you to the present and helping you to maintain your focus, in much the same way that going for a brisk walk improves children's ability to sit and focus on academic work.

DHYANA (MEDITATION): INTENSE CONTEMPLATION OF THE NATURE OF THE OBJECT OF MEDITATION, I.E, DEVOTION & MEDITATION ON THE DIVINE

The first six limbs of yoga enable you to explore applications of your ethical beliefs (the *yama* & *niyama*). These principles become engaged through movement (*asana*). You can sink into the here-and-now and breathe them deeply (*pranayama*). You can quietly listen with one sense at a time, centering yourself even in the midst of chaos (*pratyahara*). You can recover your ability to focus on one thing at a time, seeming to still the time and space around you (*dharana*). In this meditative limb (*dhyana*), you can apply all you have cultivated to the devotional object of your choice, be it a cross, a rosary, a statue of Buddha, a painting of Ganesha or Kali, or something more loosely symbolic, like a candle representing Moses' burning bush.

Yoga does not dictate your focus. You do. Each religious tradition has a myriad of symbols or icons worthy of spiritual contemplation. Pick one and contemplate. Maybe this meditation happens while maintaining a visual focal point. Maybe it's more of an auditory experience with chanting and mantras, or even the tactile devotion of prayer beads silently moving through your fingers. Whatever you choose to meditate on or with should represent the divine in a way that is meaningful to you and the faith tradition you follow. Through this meditation on familiar faces of your faith, you can access a wisdom embedded within, imprinted on your soul by one who was there when the heavens were created (Proverbs 8:27). In this place we can sit with Sophia.

Demystifying the process further, the term *dhyana*, while exotic-sounding, means simply "to think of." Moving from *dharana* to *dhyana* is like moving from the *act* of focusing to the *object* of focus. Rather than struggle with reigning the mind in and keeping it on track, *dhyana* calls us to direct all that energy at the object of our meditation. Instead of giving in to our Western proclivity to learn more about the the subject of our devotion—Jesus, Allah, Kwan Yin, Kali, etc.—we sit and endeavor to know God. To feel, hear, smell, see, and taste the divine in new ways. To encounter the wisdom of Sophia deeply and experientially.

It is at this juncture that we cease thinking about the meditation and begin to do it effortlessly—or at least with less effort than we were expending in *dharana* trying to tame our minds. I still seek the right object for my own *dhyana* practice. The cross doesn't work for me because of my sensitivity. I can't meditate on it without being drawn repeatedly to the violence that was inflicted upon it. I end up unable to maintain a peaceful state of meditation because of the images of bloodshed I'm invoking with the icon of the cross. I would rather focus on Jesus' life than his death. On his wisdom rather than his crucifixion. But what does that look like?

Maybe it doesn't look like any one object but instead feels like peace, truth, grace, forgiveness, love, or any other fruit of the spirit. Perhaps we can focus all our mental and spiritual energy on the divinely inspired attribute we feel called to that day, breathing it in, holding it within us, and releasing it into the world.

If choosing an object of divine meditation is a tough choice for me, I can imagine it's even harder for my Jewish brothers and sisters whose strict interpretation of the second commandment make choosing any representation of the divine problematic. When Moses read the words, "Thou shalt not make unto thee any graven image, or any likeness of any thing that is in heaven above..." those who follow the Jewish faith virtually abandoned the act and the art of creating divinely inspired paintings, drawings, and tapestries. I suppose most of them learned their lesson after the golden calf fiasco that caused Moses to break the original stone tablets and ascend Mt. Sinai a second time to retrieve a new set.

Evidence of subverters, driven by a deep-seated need to use art to express their spirituality, can be traced back through Jewish heritage to the Middle Ages and beyond. There is something about the beauty and symbolism of divinely inspired art that can draw us in—that can bring us closer to God. This is as true for mystical Jews as it is for contemplative types from every religion.

In *People of the Book,* Geraldine Brooks spins a fictional account of how the *Sarajeva Haggadah*—one of the earliest Jewish religious volumes to be illuminated with images—survived centuries of purges and wars thanks to people of all faiths who risked their lives to safeguard it. The words inscribed in the *Sarajeva Haggadah*, now on permanent display at the National Museum of Bosnia and Herzegovina, were not unique. They were the same words found in copies of the *Haggadah* used in Passover Seders all over the world, plentiful even in the medieval, pre-Gutenberg era of hand printing. What was worth smuggling, hiding, and lying for across centuries and borders was the language of the brightly colored images which leapt off the pages and spoke to people in a way that let them see God and their faith with new eyes. Words are not God, nor are images, but God speaks in many ways, in many tongues. Some we hear with our ears and some with our eyes. In either case, they are all just signposts pointing to a God who can be defined with neither words or images, but who chose to give us the capacity to use both in our quest for communion with the divine.

As with language, we can also stumble when we seek a visual expression of God in a feminine form, as they are few and far between. They do exist however, and can be found and contemplated regardless of your religious bent. While by no means comprehensive, here is a list of God's feminine faces—a toolbox of sorts to reach into and pull out an image on which to meditate.

SOPHIA Greek for wisdom, she is personified repeatedly in the Old Testament, yet her identify remains unclear. Some see Sophia as a deity in her own right, others as representing the Bride of Christ (Revelation 19), others as a feminine aspect of God representing wisdom (Proverbs 8 and 9), and still others as a theological concept regarding the wisdom of God.	**CHRISTIANITY/JUDAISM*** *Judaism would, obviously, use the Hebrew translation of Wisdom rather than the Greek word Sophia. Because of its nuances, you might find Wisdom expressed as khokhma (wisdom), bina (understanding), da'at (knowledge) or tvuna (another word for understanding).*	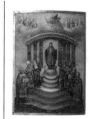
KWAN YIN Often referred to as the female Buddha, her name means, "One who hears the cries of the world."	**BUDDHISM**	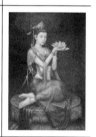
KALI One of the most fierce Hindu deities, she is paradoxically associated with both darkness and renewal.	**HINDUISM**	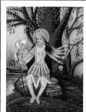
SHAKTI The personification of creative power, Shakti is known as the Great Divine Mother of Hinduism.	**HINDUISM**	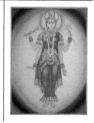

FATIMAH Daughter of the Islamic prophet Muhammad who revered her as a divine being. She is regarded by Muslims as an exemplar for men and women, as well as a symbol of The Great Mother.	**MUSLIM**	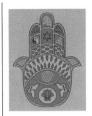
SHEKINAH Based on readings from the Talmud, represents the feminine attributes of the presence of God (Shekinah being a feminine word for dwelling or presence).	**JUDAISM** * Shekinah is often depicted as a pillar of fire or smoke, like that which led the Israelites out of Egypt.	
SHEKINAH Synonymous with the Holy Spirit, Shekinah is often associated with the New Testament term "parousia," another feminine term for divine presence.	**CHRISTIANITY** * Shekinah is imaged as the dove descending upon Mary, Jesus' mother	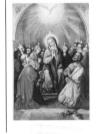

SAMADHI ("LIBERATION"): MERGING CONSCIOUSNESS WITH THE OBJECT OF MEDITATION TO REALIZE UNION WITH THE DIVINE

This idea of becoming one with God is very much in line with the mystical practices that date back to our Desert Mothers and Fathers of the fourth century who lived and breathed Psalm 46:10—"Be still and know I am God." According to modern day contemplative leader Thomas Keating, these forerunners of our faith interpreted this beloved psalm to mean "movement away from ordinary psychological awareness to the interior silence of the spiritual level of our being and beyond that, to the secrecy of the union with the Divine Indwelling within us." The experience he describes is *samadhi*. The same union is found in almost every faith tradition and, as is the case with *samadhi* in yogic philosophy, it is often the ultimate spiritual goal of the faith. The pinnacle travelers on all paths seek is this yoking of oneself to the divine.

This merging consciousness is often seen as exclusive to Eastern religions, but the truth of the matter is that the concept of uniting with the divine is equally rooted, though not always as recognized and celebrated, in Western traditions. It is a rhetorical distinction, not a theological one.

In Western Catholic theology, theosis refers to a specific and rather advanced phase of contemplation of God, not unlike the unifying experience of *samadhi* that is the eighth limb of yoga. The process of arriving at such a state, or moving toward it, involves different types of prayer which lead practitioners along purgative, illuminative, and unitive ways, known collectively as The Way.

Similarly, theosis—divinization—shows up more or less prominently in various Protestant denominations as a manifestation of divine grace. While most Protestants do not use the term theosis at all, they refer to a similar doctrine by such terms as "union with Christ" or "filled with the Holy Spirit." John Wesley, putting his unique Methodist spin on this process, developed the doctrine of sanctification which describes a state of such unity with God that sin is no longer present.

At first glance, it would appear that the Judaism's reverent fear, which precludes uttering God's name, would not be compatible with the intimacy of divine unity. However, there is evidence of divine oneness, tempered with the religion's always reverent awe of God, in the faith's mystical traditions. *The Baal* Shem *Tov's Instructions in Intercourse with God*, proclaims, "He who applies himself to the Transmission [teaching] in the fervor of cleaving to God, he makes his body the throne of the heart and the heart the throne of the spirit and the spirit the throne of the light of the indwelling glory, and he sits in the midst of the light and trembles and rejoices."

Even twelve-step programs, which are spiritual but not religious, lead to a spiritual awakening (step twelve) which is, naturally, preceded by the cultivation of a conscious contact with God (step eleven). When we are conscious of God as we go about our day, our actions and our attitude reflect that divine unity—that *samadhi,* or theosis.

In Buddhism, the meditative stages, while labeled slightly differently (*samatha, samadhi,* and *jhana*), follow much the same progression toward oneness with a divinity with a scope as all-encompassing as the universe. Paul Knitter, Professor of Theology, World Religions and Culture at Union Theological Seminary in New York City, has written a provocatively titled book, *Without Buddha I Could Not Be a Christian.* Based on his integration of Buddhist thought and practice into his Catholic faith, he explores his "double belonging" and describes how his Zen practice helped him through his struggles with his Christian faith. I am struck again that there are many paths—often intersecting, crisscrossing each other over and over—on the spiritual roads we all travel toward salvation, heaven, and enlightenment.

If quieting the mind so that we can focus on spiritual matters is our universal goal, why is it so difficult for most of us? The idea of *samadhi* is affirmed in many faith traditions; however the concept of being still—of doing nothing—and letting God come to us, dwell in us, is far removed from our modern sensibilities. Those operating within Western religious paradigms resist the concept of meditation and experience the obstacles to it even more acutely than our Buddhist sisters and brothers who outlined these five hindrances to a state of deep meditation:

1. Sensual Desire: Craving for pleasure to the senses.
2. Anger or ill-will: Feelings of malice directed toward others.
3. Sloth-torpor or boredom: Half-hearted action with little or no concentration.
4. Restlessness-worry: The inability to calm the mind.
5. Doubt: Lack of conviction or trust.

The first hindrance, our craving for sensual desires, would be those thoughts that tell us we could meditate better if only we had a comfier bench, a steaming cup of tea, or warm socks on our feet. These misleading thoughts are the "if onlys." I could meditate contentedly, "if only..." In life, this leads us to the mistaken belief that we'd be happy "if only...".

The next hindrance, stemming from anger or ill-will, is made up of thoughts that boomerang back at us from earlier in the day, the week or even the year. Undealt with resentments will continue coming back to haunt us if we don't find a way to process them and let them go.

The third hindrance, boredom, is exacerbated by the trend toward constant connection among 21st century Americans. *Samadhi* requires such a complete disconnect from external and internal stimuli that it blows in opposition to the prevailing winds of the culture.

Boredom breeds restlessness, the fourth obstacle that stands between us and *samadhi*. An inability to just be. Worry, companion to restlessness, is what the mind grasps at when it can't bear to do nothing.

Our worry grows out of the fact that we aren't trusting God or our Higher Power to take care of our needs—the fifth and final hindrance. We are operating within the false bravado of a culture that espouses independence above all. Our country was founded on it, and it's a wonderful thing—in moderation.

If you're in need of an antidote, flip to Matthew 6:28-30: "And why be anxious about clothing? Learn a lesson from the way the wildflowers grow. They don't work; they don't spin. Yet I tell you, not even Solomon in full splendor was arrayed like one of these. If God can clothe in such splendor the grasses of the field, which bloom today and are thrown on the fire tomorrow, won't God do so much more for you—you who have such little faith?" Consider setting a vase of fresh flowers near your meditation area to remind you of how beautifully God will adorn you if you let Her.

There is no way to enter a state of *samadhi* with any one of these loitering in your head. How do we rid our mind of these unwelcome intruders? Climb back down a couple of limbs. The answer is sure to lie in one of them. Go out and perform a random act of kindness (*yama* & *niyama*), incorporate some breathing exercises into your meditation time (*pranayama*), get up and focus on some body-expanding *asanas*. Just maybe your mind will follow.

UNITING YOGA'S LIMBS

Virtually every type of yoga class offered in the United States is a Hatha yoga class, so that label alone will not tell you much about a class. Fifteenth century Indian sage Yogi Swatmarama coined the term Hatha yoga, and it has since come to be associated with all forms of asana practice. While classes that go by that name may differ widely in specific content and format, what brands them as Hatha yoga is their focus on the two physical limbs of the Raja yoga system—*asana* (physical postures) and *pranayama* (breath). According to Swatmarama, the practice of Hatha yoga is "a stairway to the height of Raja yoga," preparing the practitioner for the more subtle practices of meditation and increased conscious contact with God through the vigorous physical practices.

Hatha means forceful in Sanskrit. It is this forceful physical work that, according to Patanjali, allows for the subsequent mental, emotional, and spiritual release. The body learns the lessons first, then the mind and heart follow.

Yoga's physical, mental, and spiritual practices can be used as a path to the divine within any faith tradition, leading us to sacred wisdom. To Sophia. Awareness and practice of yoga's universal principles can bring about a subtle alignment with spiritual seekers around us who may have chosen different religious roads but are heading in the same direction. Looking at the ways we are alike in no way diminishes the strength of each of our own, distinct belief systems. His Holiness The Dalai Lama was a living example of this precept when he agreed to provide a Buddhist perspective on the teachings of Jesus at an interfaith gathering in the mid-1990s. While reading *The Good Heart*, the book that resulted from the historic address, I was struck by his humility and respect for a belief system different from his own. In an age where it seems we are all fighting to be right, hearing him speak with such reverence on the teachings of another faith was nothing short of awe-inspiring.

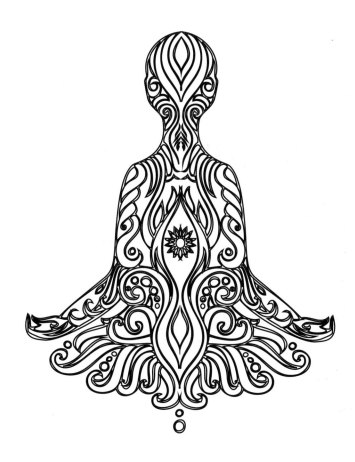

CHAPTER 3

Recovering Yoga

"YOGA IS FOR ALL. TO LIMIT YOGA TO THE
BOUNDARIES OF ONE NATION IS THE DENIAL OF
UNIVERSAL CONSCIOUSNESS."
—B.K.S. IYENGAR

Many people within the Judeo-Christian faith communities have seen yoga and other forms of Eastern meditation as a threat to traditional Western religions. Conversely, those of the Hindu faith sometimes want to claim yoga as their proprietary practice. But nobody owns yoga. The contemplative, meditative practices of Judaism and early Christianity have much in common with yogic spirituality. Seeing them together, it appears that we in the West are not discovering yoga, but recovering part of our spiritual heritage. A part of our heritage that uses forgotten mystical practices as a doorway to Sophia, God's wisdom.

In what is perhaps the first published account of yoga from a Christian perspective, Father J.M. DeChanet, a French Benedictine, presents yoga as a means of encouraging a return to contemplative practices in order to counteract the tension of the modern world, saying:

> Christ came in the first place so that this 'creature of God' within us, concealed under a human complex, bruised and torn by original sin, should flower and open out in its full beauty and wealth of talent. Any ascetic discipline that works towards this works, in fact, hand in hand with grace, and that is why I have roundly stated that a yoga that calms the senses, pacifies the soul, and frees certain intuitive or affective powers in us can be of inestimable service to the West. It can make people into true Christians, dynamic and open (*Christian Yoga*, 1960).

Those sentiments are still considered radical today, as leaders within various Christian denominations continue to denounce yoga as incompatible with Christianity or even demonic, but they were positively revolutionary when Father DeChanet revealed himself as a Benedictine yogi more than fifty years ago.

A *Time* magazine cover story, published in July 1960, gave DeChanet the high-visibility platform he needed to introduce the concept of a Christian yogi to Westerners hungry for a way to express their spirituality in the midst of the counter-cultural rumblings that were about to revolutionize their world—like it or not. He described the spiritual benefits of yoga in ways that made sense to those intrigued by the practice, even using language familiar to church-going Christians. The Christian yogi, he claimed, had made his [or her] body into a faithful servant. "You order it (and it obeys) to help you to practise fully even virtues as great as faith, hope and Christian charity."

What Dechanet set out to do when he first began to practice yoga in his early forties was not to turn it into something Christian, but to use it for Christian purposes. His main purpose was to harmonize the three elements in humanity which the early church designated as *anima* (the body and its functions), *animus* (the reasoning, analytical mind), and *spiritus* (the loving soul, yearning toward the Divine).

Twenty-five years later, Reverend Albrecht Frenz of Stuttgart, Germany, continued this melding of Eastern practice with Western religion when he extolled the virtues of yoga, saying, "The practice of Yoga makes available the peace and quietness of spirit which enables the Holy Ghost to become more active within the soul." In the introduction, Bishop C.S. Sundaresan says:

> "There is a lot of prejudice against Yoga; it is mainly due, in most cases, to lack of correct information and wholesome knowledge of the disciplines of Yoga which can be appropriated by any religious practitioner for reaping the benefits one's religion can give. Most people practice Yoga for physical and mental well-being. In so far, it is good; but it is not enough. They must go beyond them into the spiritual realm with faith and perseverance, trusting in God's grace."

How did Father DeChanet, Reverend Frenz, and Bishop Sundaresan come to believe that yoga is a spiritual discipline that can serve seekers of many faiths? It certainly wasn't spelled out for them in sacred texts or their religious traditions. Or was it? To answer those questions, we will have to go back to the beginning of the story. Back to yoga's revered sage Patanjali and Christianity's messiah, Jesus Christ.

POINTING THE WAY

While Patanjali is thought to have lived several hundred years after Christ's death, Indian sages—called *Siddhas*—had been practicing yogic philosophy, including the eight limbs of yoga, for thousands of years before Jesus appeared on the scene. Patanjali, it turns out, didn't create the eight limbs, he simply wrote them down. His seminal writing provided a much-needed record of this spiritual heritage that had been transmitted strictly via oral tradition. The written tradition that emerged from this period of Indian spirituality is today referred to as the *Upanishads*.

These Indian *Siddhas*, who would have been Jesus' contemporaries, were working within much the same paradigm as Jesus and his early followers, most likely without ever having contact with the historical figure of Jesus. In his book on this subject, *The Wisdom of Jesus and the Yoga Siddhas*, yogi and wisdom scholar Marshall Govindan provides a fascinating look at the similarities between the *Siddhas*' teachings and Jesus'. Five parallels stand out to me.

Teaching Style... Both Jesus and the *Siddhas* taught in paradoxes, articulating profound truths through simple parables and poetry that even the illiterate masses could understand, at least at a basic level. The delivery may have been simplified to ensure wide assimilation of the message, but there was a deeper, almost hidden, meaning in both traditions, accessible to those who were still and quiet enough hear it speaking to them.

Inner Wisdom... Both pointed to the fact that the real temple, the destination for true transformation, was not a physical structure that imposed religion from the outside, but rather our own inner soul experiences. Like Jesus, the *Siddhas* condemned idol worship and promoted true spiritual wisdom over the knowledge gleaned in the temples. Though rooted in Hinduism, the *Siddhas* did not extoll the virtues of any of the myriad of Hindu deities. The discovery of this inner wisdom is the Sophia experience that can manifest in any soul that seeks it.

Intention... Neither the *Siddhas* nor Jesus set out to create a new religion. Their words and actions made this abundantly clear, though we often forget this when we trace our religious roots and end up at their feet. Both of them were very much speakers of spiritual truth, not organizers of religious institutions.

Forgiveness & Detachment... These are two different names for a similar concept advocated by both Jesus and the *Siddhas*. Govindan makes the point that both require a "dispassion," a letting go of what we're comfortable with and embracing what might feel foreign to us. In order to forgive, for example, we must let go of our wounded ego just like the father in Jesus' parable of the prodigal son. The father had to detach from the initial betrayal he felt from his son's abandonment. That detachment was part of the process of forgiving.

The Kingdom Within Us... Both the *Siddhas* and Jesus based their teachings on this key concept. In Matthew, Mark, and Luke, we get the most undiluted version of Jesus' message. In these books, we hear that the "Kingdom of Heaven" is within us over and over again. This differs markedly from other Biblical sources of Jesus' teachings—like the Epistles of Paul and the Gospel of John—which focus on Jesus' mission and person. Interestingly, the two outwardly focused books are widely considered to be interpolations or accounts in which unknown sources attribute quotes directly to Jesus, while the inward focus is attributed more directly to him. Using different terminology, the *Siddhas* describe this inner kingdom as Absolute Being, Consciousness, or Bliss. Contrary to our Western understanding, these terms do not refer to self-created states of being, but to a personal realization of what God already sees in us and is already doing in us. In her contemplative classic, *The Wisdom Jesus*, Episcopal priest Cynthia Bourgeault perfectly captures the fallacy in the typical interpretation of The Kingdom of Heaven, saying, "You don't die into it, you awaken into it."

Through the practice of yoga, I have recovered aspects of my faith that were there in the earliest rumblings of creation, shaped by "a master craftswoman ever at play by God's side" (Proverbs 8:30). I unearthed them not in a temple, but on a mat—a spot unconsecrated by any religion. I learned I could detach from the chaos of the world through utterances as simple as the syllable "ohm," and moments filled only with the sound of my own breath. I stumbled upon the kingdom of heaven. Sophia was there, and she pointed the way.

Language is key to creating or breaking down our understanding of one another. Just as patriarchal language can alienate female or egalitarian readers, language associated with Eastern mysticism—terms like "Bliss" or "Absolute Being"—can fall on deaf ears when spoken to Western Christians who may have forgotten about the koanical nature of Jesus' teachings. When we stop to ponder paradoxes like the need to become child-like to enter the kingdom of heaven (Matthew 18:2-4), "Bliss" and

81

"Absolute Being" begin to make sense. As does Sophia who was "at play everywhere in God's domain, delighting to be with the children of humanity" (Proverbs 8:31).

There are some remarkable groups dedicated to bridging these gaps in language, imagery, and practice. In the case of women in the church, Christians for Biblical Equality is at the forefront, providing literature, speakers, and other resources to help individuals and institutions work through the process of dropping old gender-based limitations often rooted in language.

In 1942, Koinonia (Greek for communion)—an intentional Christian community which shares its roots with Habitat for Humanity—was founded by Clarence Jordan in Americus, Georgia. Since that time, it has consistently, and often controversially, lived out Jesus' radical call to discipleship by confronting racism, militarism, and materialism with its commitment to:

1.   Treat all human beings with dignity and justice.
2.   Choose love over violence.
3.   Share all possessions and live simply.
4.   Be stewards of the land and its natural resources.

Innocuous enough in theory, these practices caused quite a stir packaged as they were in the form of a commune plucked down in the middle of the South where people of all ethnicities lived and worked side-by-side, even before the transformation of the Civil Rights movement began.

Similarly, today the D. L. Dykes, Jr. Foundation connects modern Christians to their spiritual roots through their Faith & Reason initiative, bringing speakers, literature, and audio/video recordings to contemplative seekers. In a newsletter re-cap of their recent gathering to discuss Jesus and his parables, they articulated their commitment to speaking the truth in a context that invokes the truth of the historical Jesus:

The language we use about faith is critical. The words we select are crucial. It matters very much that our claims about historical Jesus are grounded not only in a sacred text, but also that they are grounded in

82

the stones and on the epitaphs of the first century. To authentically participate in Christian tradition means to take seriously what was going on in the world when historical Jesus resisted the domination system of his own day and encouraged and insisted on non-violent alternatives to the way empire civilizations do business on any given day. Our words, our claims matter greatly. We create our words; our words create us. We make our claims about what is historical and authentic about historical Jesus. And these claims we make about historical Jesus surely claim us.

Profoundly articulating the need for recovering the energy, the faith, and the wisdom put forth by Jesus while he was here on Earth, this statement reminds us that Jesus was never one to follow the letter of the law, but was spirit-led. Ironically, if we focus too much on our sacred text, as it has been handed down and interpreted over the past 2,000+ years, we are missing much of Jesus' message. We end up knowing about Jesus, but we don't know him. To get the full picture, we have to travel back and study those ancient stones and epitaphs, running our fingers over them, breathing them in and walking in the footsteps of the Jesus who was present with them. This process expands the limited view we get from the translation of those texts that were deemed worthy of canonization some 170 to 400 years after Jesus' human form left us.

Reconciling the 2,000-year-old practices and conceptions of Jesus with that of modern day Christianity, contemplative author Cynthia Bourgeault ends a 2004 lecture with this explanation, "The roots of Christian mysticism are not really in historical time; they are in the Kingdom. And Mysticism seen in this light is not an individualized, subjective experience of God. It is the tie-rod connecting the worlds." True to form, it sounds a bit like a koan, drawing you in, raising questions and leaving you to ponder them.

Traditionally used in Zen Buddhism, a koan—a paradox to be meditated upon—is given by a teacher to a student as a way to help them access spiritual insights. Unlike linear Western inquiry which seeks logical conclusions, koans require an intuitive approach using lateral, rather than critical, thinking. In Matthew 10:39, Jesus crafts the perfectly paradoxical koan, saying, "You who have found your life will lose it, and you who lose your life for my sake will find it."

Because we know little of the logistical details of Jesus' life in the "missing years" between his recorded teaching in the temple at age twelve and the beginning of his mission at age thirty, there is no way to know for certain who he came in contact with and was influenced by during this period. Many have posited a plausible connection between Jesus and the Essene community, a Jewish sect to which John the Baptist may have belonged.

In any case, while Jesus was a master who needed no spiritual direction, it is clear that he chose to live in community, and to steep himself in the teachings and practices of spiritual seekers around him. The way he participated in this experience of community was not typical of a learned priest. He directed without the hierarchical, authoritarian approach which removed most leaders from their followers. Bourgeault proposes the role of Sufi sheik as most analogous to Jesus' work as a spiritual master, noting the threefold nature of the sheik's function: wisdom teacher, spiritual elder, and channel for the direct transmission of blessing. All roles Jesus assumed in his time on earth.

DEFINING THE WAY

Mystic traditions, by their very nature, embrace the unknowable. Even so, a means of defining what that shrouded divinity looks like in day-to-day life can provide a spiritual structure, a loosely sketched road map for contemplatives in need of grounding.

Spiritual definition is a slippery creature. At best, it points us in the right direction. Idling in neutral, it's somewhat arbitrary. And when used to repress and control, it's downright harmful. A quest to possess our faith or contain God through definition can cause consternation. But there is another way. One that takes a mystical approach and seeks spiritual wisdom—Sophia—facilitated by the practical parameters found in yoga. Teresa of Avila says, "One knows God in oneself, and knows oneself in God." The knowing is permanent and real, the rest—the dogma, the rules, the religious rhetoric—we can let go when it conflicts with or inhibits our experience of God.

As we seek to put words—to give a fitting name—to the road that leads us from ourselves to something more, we find a harmony exists between the yogic and Christian paths. The Eight Limbs of Yoga, it turns out, are remarkably similar to The Way, a little-known spiritual path laid out by 5th century theologian Pseudo-Dionysius, often called the father of Christian mysticism. Both cover three areas of spiritual growth: wisdom, ethical conduct, and mental development.

Christianity's way and yoga's eight limbs both begin with ethics, move through wisdom, and conclude by defining mental constructs. Mental development, in this context, does not refer to the development of mental abilities or faculties. Rather, it is the melding of one's mind with the wisdom and ethics already absorbed. The aim of these spiritual blueprints—in both yoga and Christianity—is the development of a single-pointed vision of the soul. Sophia, representing God's wisdom at work within, embodies this single point.

A comparison of the two systems, broken out into these three areas, looks like this:

EIGHT LIMBS

Ethical Conduct (1st and 2nd Limbs)
>   *Yama* (universal morality)
>   *Niyama* (personal observances)

Wisdom (3rd - 5th Limbs)
>   *Asanas* (body postures)
>   *Pranayama* (breathing exercises)
>   *Pratyahara* (control of senses)

Mental Development (6th - 8th Limbs)
>   *Dharana* (concentration)
>   *Dhyana* (meditation)
>   *Samadhi* (liberation)

THE WAY

Ethical Conduct
>   Purgative Way

Wisdom
>   Illuminative Way

Mental Development
>   Unitive Way

85

Those with a Catholic background, might find these terms as familiar as rosary beads worn down by decades of fingering. Christians not raised in the Catholic Church, may find them just as foreign as yoga's eight limbs. I find it interesting that these parallel paths come from the mystics within their respective traditions. Not from the high priests or formal leaders, but from those who yearned to find a way to encounter God, to lay out practices and ways to lead others into a divine presence. Into what one medieval mystic called the cloud of unknowing in a classic contemplative text by the same name.

These luminaries were not apologetics interested in answering all the questions. Rather, they were seekers interested in questioning all the answers. Implicit to the perpetual state of unknowing in contemplative traditions is the ability to live in a place where there is no need to know and to name God as anything other than the embodiment of the divine. Because of this receptiveness, there is room for God to become more than a father figure. In contemplative contexts, meaning is sought beneath the surface of sacred texts and the experience of God is multi-faceted. Leaving behind liturgical limits; God surfaces in a majestic sunset, parades divine beauty through our lives, and rests as Sophia in the stillness of our souls.

A maternal beckoning is a hallmark of both The Way and the Eight Limbs. While neither is matriarchal by design, they are both inclusive of the feminine voice. Both contemplatives and yogis hear and heed the call of Mother God where others may turn a deaf ear to her, believing that only Father God speaks truth.

St. Thomas Aquinas (1225-1275)—though firmly rooted in Aristotle's erroneous biological presuppositions that made his view of women less-than-favorable—was, nevertheless, a proponent of the mystical path that came to be known as The Way. He describes the three-part journey as such:

The first duty which is incumbent on man is to give up sin and resist concupiscence, which are opposed to charity; this belongs to beginners, in whose hearts charity is to be nursed and cherished lest it be corrupted. The second duty of man is to apply his energies chiefly to advance in virtue; this belongs to those who are making progress and who are principally concerned that charity may be increased and strengthened in them. The third endeavor and pursuit of man should be to rest in God and enjoy Him; and this belongs to the perfect who desire to be dissolved and to be with Christ.

The first phase of The Way, the Purgative State, encompasses the same spiritual growth as the the *yama* and *niyama* of yoga, prescriptive guidance that helps spiritual seekers put divine commandments into practice. This is Spirituality 101 in both traditions. Both start with refining the most fundamental aspects of one's self, that is the behavior that's outwardly exhibited and the internal impulses that drive it. This initial way of approaching faith is designed, as its name implies, to purge unwanted behaviors from one's life. The focus of the Purgative Way is to strengthen and nourish virtues (*niyama*), while endeavoring to resist temptations (*yama*).

The Illuminative Way actively works to cultivate that still, quiet space within. It is where we can begin to sense Sophia at work. This Christian path to wisdom mirrors yoga's wisdom limbs of *asana* (body postures), *pranayama* (breathing exercises) and *pratyahara* (control of the senses). Moving closer to union with God, this state finds us abiding in God's presence, surrounded by the contemplative tasks of silence, recollection, retirement, simplicity, and right intention. All the same attributes we seek to access via our yogic *asanas*, breathing and sensory practices.

It is at intersections like this that we begin to see the synchronicity between Christianity's faith path and a yogic one. If we have that single-pointed vision Jesus talks about (Luke 11:34), it really is all one path with no dualism splintering us off into different directions or segmenting our life into compartments. Likewise, the Illuminative Way is clearly not one of hibernation, where we withdraw from the world, creating a spiritual cocoon within which we draw closer to God by retreating from our callings in this world. Indeed, the tension and the beauty lies in reconciling these inner and outer worlds, creating the illuminative state's goal of "a most holy union with God."

From this holy union, we are swept into the Unitive Way which corresponds with the sixth through eighth limbs of yoga, *dharana* (concentration), *dhyana* (meditation), and *samadhi* (liberation). Both the Unitive

Way and yoga seek to yoke us to God. St. Paul describes this union when he says: "But whoever is joined to Christ becomes one spirit with Christ" (I Corinthians 6:17). This is precisely what we do in the final three limbs of yoga. The three yogic distinctions simply articulate the nuances of the overarching union espoused in the Unitive Way.

Debating which spiritual framework—the Eight Limbs, The Way, or some other comparable path—is more effective is a bit like arguing about which came first, the chicken or the egg? The answer is really quite arbitrary. It's the process that matters. God doesn't care about our terminology or give demerits for doing spiritual work out of order.

This is something I need to remind myself whenever I am tempted to make religion or doctrine my God. If it was written down and ordained by a human like me, it is merely the sharing of someone else's fallible ideas. While the paths we are examining are all deeply profound and instructive to spiritual seekers, each is merely a chronicle of one person or one group's experience with God. Their road map for traveling the road to commune with divinity. The day-to-day guidance I receive directly from Sophia usually looks much less linear, arriving in unofficial, unorthodox packages that look more like spring leaves or a ball-of-fire sunrise bursting over the horizon. It sounds like a flowing brook or children's laughter, sometimes disguising its voice as a casual comment whose wisdom is revealed only in God's good time. It feels like a book falling open in my lap, randomly, it would seem, except that the words spilling out seem to be written just for me.

Grasping this strength and the corresponding limitation in their own faith tradition, Christian contemplatives have adopted intentional practices that date back centuries to help move them along their own spiritual path. In an humble admission, Father Keating acknowledges, "The purgative and unitive ways are well differentiated, but the path from one to the other does not seem to adequately address the physical, psychological, and spiritual obstacles that hinder the process, especially unconscious motivation and habits of negative behavior." It appears what's missing is the "how to" of illumination, a way to achieve what the Illuminative Way imparts, bridging the gap between the commencement and fulfillment of a spiritual journey.

To fill this void, Keating and others have established intentional practices through which to engage their faith, anchoring them to a direct experience with God. Discovering these sacred keys provides entrance to "the inner room" Jesus describes in Matthew 6:6. In the Judeo-Christian tradition, we are told to "be still and know I am God," but we are not given instruction on how to still ourselves enough to know this in more than a superficial, intellectual way. Cerebral exercises will not bridge this gap. Experiential practices—ones that show us rather than tell us—can transport us spiritually, so much so that we may smell the salty air of the Dead Sea while tracing the sandy footprints of our Desert Mothers and Fathers beckoning us to follow them.

PRACTICING THE WAY
"A certain brother went to Abba Moses in Scete, and asked him for a good word. And the elder said to him: Go, sit in your cell, and your cell will teach you everything." – Thomas Merton (Wisdom of the Desert)

Such a simple prescription for accessing that Kingdom of Heaven Jesus so often referenced. Simple in the directive—"sit." Like the most basic command we teach our dogs, and reminiscent of the very first yoga *asana* we learn, *"namastiti,"* or simple seated pose. This "seat" we take in *asana* practice or in the contemplative posture Moses advocates, prepares us for meditation and eventually to accessing that elusive kingdom within. Simple, too, in its setting. Could there be a more austere space than a cell? The concept of a cell conjures up extreme sparsity, visions of a life lived unencumbered by any of the trappings that complicate our existence.

We have a cultural propensity to hold so tightly to our possessions, both literal and emotional, that we can't reach out and fully grasp all God is offering us. Our space—in opposition to the starkness of the cell Moses describes—is so cluttered that it's hard to see the sacred under all the stuff we've piled around us. The yogic *yama* of non-possessiveness (*aparigraha*) and Jesus' teachings remind us that we are not defined by what we own. In his seminal words on the topic, Jesus lays all of the false worth we place in ownership to rest saying, "Don't store up earthly treasures for yourselves, which moths and rust destroy and thieves can break

89

in and steal" (Matthew 6:19). The Message's modern translation drives the point home, adding, "It's obvious, isn't it? The place where your treasure is, is the place you will most want to be, and end up being."

Despite how obvious this truth seems to be, we often have difficulty carrying it out in our lives. The theory, while intellectually palatable, remains difficult to embrace in day-to-day living. To discover why, we need to delve into the mind-set that creates such disconnects for us.

First, there's the interesting etymological kinship of the words mother and matter, both derived from the Latin root *mater*. Without even being consciously aware of this linguistic connection, we often try to fill the gaping mother holes in our spiritual lives with matter. That explains our consumption-induced clutter. While intellectually we know we can't buy back the Mother God that's been lost, our subconscious tries to fill those hungry places in our soul with whatever's available. And there's no shortage of stuff! Until we stop defining God as exclusively male and give ourselves free reign to explore a God that has no use for limiting gender stereotypes, we will find ourselves trying and failing to grasp a God who's our mother, our father, and so much more.

We need to be empty in spirit—free from unnecessary dogma and preconceived notions about God—if we are to experience God for ourselves on a meaningful level. There is a well-know Zen parable that perfectly expresses this need for receptiveness in spiritual seekers. A student, interviewing with the spiritual master under which he hopes to study, prattles on about his accomplishments and opinions. During this monologue, the master calmly pours tea until the student's cup is overflowing. Finally the student, jolted out of his self-centered reverie, exclaims, "Stop pouring! The cup is full." The teacher replies, "Yes, and so are you. How can I possibly teach you?"

Second, there's the unnatural separation we impose on our world—between us and God, us and other people, and between the various facets of our lives. Eastern traditions call this dualism. If you are feeling fractured, disconnected or otherwise unwhole, dualism may be at work in your life. Insidious, it creeps up on us, erecting walls that cordon off the parts of life deemed sacred, leaving the rest to languish, unconnected to the divine. Jesus had a thing or two to say about avoiding this crazy-making paradigm.

His seminal statement of non-duality was his assertion that "For Abba and I are one" (John 10:30). Devoid of separation and judgement, the proclamation embodies the unity we seek through our yoga—compelling us to reconcile the disjointed pieces of our lives and our souls. Duality, as a pervasive construct, runs so deeply through Christianity that we often fail to see it at work, setting up oppositional forces that thwart our spiritual growth. We end up in a black and white world full of good and evil, heaven and hell, salvation and damnation. We idolize and vilify, setting in motion a pattern of placing things on pedestals and running in fear lest they fall on us.

Why do you think Rob Bell's latest book, *Love Wins*, stirred up so much controversy? Not the title. There are not many who would argue against love. The subtitle—*Heaven, Hell & the Fate of Every Person Who Ever Lived*—is the hornet's nest. In the book—which suggests that the gospel's news is, perhaps, not so good if it condemns the bulk of the world's people to hell—he refuses to accept the duality inherent in the traditional Christian view of Heaven and Hell. Good and Evil. Saved and Damned. He poses the forbidden question many were afraid to ask, "Isn't God bigger than all this?" And he answers a resounding, "Yes."

The imbedded "us vs. them" mentality is fueled by a dualistic focus on garnering ourselves a place among the saved, rather than being a saving grace for the world we're in. Phrases like "God's Chosen People" and "Children of God" come loaded with the assumption that some are in and some are out. Likewise, referring to God in possessive terms, "our God," (as it's belted out in the contemporary hymn by the same name) perpetuates the myth that God is ownable and exclusive to one particular group. I cringe whenever I hear that song with its subtle attempt to lay claim to a divinity that flows out in all directions, refusing to be dammed.

Using that as a starting point for our faith almost assures those fissures in our collective consciousness will remain, for they cannot possibly be healed as long as we are operating within a system based on laws of exclusion and inclusion. In his ever-accessible wisdom, Dr. Seuss tells us the story of the Sneeches enticed into an unending cycle of status-seeking by a slick salesman offering to apply or remove the status-laden stars from their bellies. Soon, Sneeches are being branded and unbranded at breakneck speed. As long as we are parading about as star-bellied Sneeches, while looking askance (in pity or derision) at those who have "no stars upon thars," we are doomed to miss the single-pointed vision Jesus was trying to impart to us.

He articulates the impact of a non-dual consciousness in Luke 11:34, saying, "The light of the body is the eye: therefore when thine eye is single, thy whole body also is full of light; but when [thine eye] is evil, thy body also [is] full of darkness" (KJV). I chose the King James version for that particular verse because I like the specificity of the word "single" to describe the state we should seek for our eyes, the single-pointed vision to which we aspire. Other versions speak of the eye being "well" or "sound," neither of which provides as much guidance to us.

Bourgeault further contributes to our understanding of The Kingdom of Heaven, reminding us that "it's not later, it's lighter." This is an echo of Jesus directive to live in the present: "The reign of God does not come in a visible way. You can't say, 'See, here it is!' or 'There it is!' No—look: the reign of God is already in your midst" (Luke 17:20-21).

Yoga's eight limbs are practical steps that can create a space where we can begin to see God's kingdom both enveloping us and residing within us. The wisdom found in this place of stillness is Sophia. In this yogic worldview, universality replaces duality. Within this construct everyone is a child of God, and everything is sacred. Religions, including Christianity and Judaism, are not only compatible with this way of thinking, but actually flourish as faith—moving, breathing, and resting—becomes deeply assimilated into the rhythm of life.

The late Father Jacques Dupuis, renowned Belgian theologian who spent many years as a professor of a Jesuit-run seminary in Delhi, applied the concept of *advaita*, a monastic school of thought within Hinduism, to Christianity. He saw *advaita*, literally translated as non-duality, as a way to achieve a single-pointed mind-set as a follower of Jesus. In *Christ-Consciousness and Advaitic Experience*, he explains that if Jesus' religious experience consists of his human awareness of being one with the Father, so should ours. This, he claims, is Christian *advaita*.

We can choose to expand our own *advaita* to include unity with a God whose boundaries extend beyond the role of father. When we are open to seeing God unbridled by our own conceptions, we can begin to experience *advaita* in unexpected places. As we behold God our Mother, hearken back to the Latin root of both mother and matter (mater) with which we started this deconstruction. Our challenge is to try not to fill ourselves up with its culturally pervasive derivative—materialism, but to be led instead by our spiritual mother—Sophia.

Yoga can return us to a place where we can experience spiritual mothering through practices rooted in Christianity's ancient wisdom tradition. We are transported back to a simpler time when Jesus' teachings were mediated by a few hundred years rather than a few thousand. To a time when people didn't ask each other, "What would Jesus do?" because he had not been so long gone that his voice had faded from our collective memory. Elders still spoke about his divine humanity within a tapestry of oral tradition that mingled folklore with family stories in which Jesus and his miracles were vibrant threads.

We have a universal need to weave these threads into our own lives, to graft ourselves to the life-giving vine Jesus talks about in John 15:5. It is this earnest quest for true divine connection that moves us beyond the rote recitations and rambling confessions to which we are accustomed, sending us to quiet, still places that can only be found when we, ourselves, are quiet and still. There are practices which took root in Christianity as the Eight Limbs were spreading over Hinduism, offering us the shade of spiritual formation and renewal should we just sit with them a while. Stemming from Christian tradition and thought—sometimes even from Jesus' own lips—they bear a remarkable resemblance to the practices we discovered in our journey through yoga's eight limbs.

While the two paths weave, crisscross and veer apart, their intention and the resulting destination are identical. Literally translated, yoga's cumulative state of *samadhi* means to acquire integration, wholeness or truth. The eighth limb of yoga by the same name calls us to realize union with the divine. Startlingly similar, Christianity's Unitive Way is the union with God by love and the actual experience and exercise of that love. So what does that look like, this journey to the Unitive Way? Beginning with the earliest Christian experience following Jesus' example of contemplation, let's unearth some tools that may have escaped our attention or become pedantic traditions rather than meaningful practices.

HESYCHASM: OUR FERTILE GROUND

Hesychasm is the process—achieved via a myriad of contemplative practices—of retiring inward by ceasing to register the senses, in order to achieve direct, experiential knowledge of God. Indeed, very reminiscent of our journey through the eight limbs. Its impetus within Christianity is Jesus' admonition to "go into your closet to pray."

Hesychasm—from the Greek *heschia* meaning "quiet" or "the silent life"—is the most basic and original mystical expression of Eastern Christianity. Before we insert our natural dualistic perspective, separating and dismissing Eastern Christianity and its spiritual disciplines as unlike our Western Christianity, let's remember that Christianity is innately Eastern, not Western. We Westernized it to suit our own cultural needs.

The fundamental difference in Eastern and Western Christianity lies not in variations of core beliefs, but in our approach to those beliefs. In the West, we intellectualize. The Eastern approach is more experiential. Bourgeault traces this approach back to Western Christianity's Roman lineage, noting that "the two chief earmarks of the Roman filter are that it tends to confuse unity with uniformity and puts a high priority on order and authority." Those cultural biases shaped not only our religion, but our conceptions of God.

Numerous scholars have attributed the divergent world views within Christianity to the paths of Jesus' original apostles. Paul (and perhaps Peter at some point, though that is debatable) went West into the Roman Empire, establishing the tradition of Christianity that has come to be seen by those of us in the West as representative of Christianity as a whole. In truth, it is but one manifestation of it.

A holistic vision of Christianity's establishment following Jesus' ascension looks much different than the straight and narrow path we typically envision leading from Palestine directly to Rome.

Tangents from this road to the Greco-Roman world include a route, begun by one or more of the original apostles, which headed southwest to Africa, across the Gibraltar Strait and the coast of France, landing in the Celtic realm of the British Isles. Other apostles moved east into Persia, India and China, naturally cultivating a Christianity with Eastern undertones. Still other apostles were called to stay firmly planted in the Middle East, giving

94

life to a Christian culture in what is today a largely Islamic area including Iraq, Syria, and Turkey. Bourgeault surmises, "All of these energy streams flowing out from the Jesus event had their own unique flavors—and they are very different from the flavor we're used to in our own stream."

This radiating scheme seems a more likely scenario than the one-pronged approach so often presented to us. Because St. Thomas was purported to have reached India before Peter or Paul reached Rome, the first sowing of Christian culture outside of its Middle Eastern origins would have been Mediterranean or Asian in nature. I agree with Matus that "the Gospel is at home in the East as much as in the West." Because it is indigenous to the East, maybe more so. Yoga, then, can serve as a bridge to the lost Eastern heritage of the earliest expressions of Christianity.

There are many theological terms to describe the distinction between Eastern and Western approaches to religion. Prophetic (religion of the word) vs. mystical (religion of divine unity) and kataphatic (defining God through symbols, words, liturgy, etc.) vs. apophatic (directly experiencing the mystery of God) are just two you may encounter. Though we naturally place them in a mutually exclusive context (even linguistically as I demonstrated with the use of "versus" in each pair) they are not meant to exist in opposition, but in communion with one another.

To create a holistic faith experience, we must incorporate both approaches—both sides of the same coin—to engage our entire being. In addition to this melding of interior and exterior realms there is a deeper and more fundamental difference in the Eastern and Western views. It lies in our basic conception of Jesus and the role he plays in our faith journeys.

Soteriology, upon which all Western theology is based, relates to Jesus primarily as a savior (from the Greek "soter" meaning savior), while Eastern theology espouses sophiology (from the Greek "sophia" meaning wisdom), interpreting him as a life-giver, based on the understanding of early Aramaic-speaking Christians (including Jesus) for whom there was no word for salvation or savior.

As with other spiritual dichotomies, the truth lies not in the opposition of the two, but in their union. It's found in that place where we can truly claim Jesus as our savior and our purest source of wisdom. In abandoning dualistic thought, we embrace our own spiritual truth.

HESYCHASTIC PRAYER: THE JESUS PRAYER

This sophiological understanding combined with the hesychasm of the burgeoning monastic movements of early Eastern Christianity formed the fertile spiritual ground that yields many of the contemplative forms of worship still used today. The hesychastic method of prayer, also known as the Jesus prayer, is one early example. Though *hesychasm*—by its very nature—involves silence and stillness, by far the most popular form of hesychastic prayer involves speaking. Not just a word or two, but the repetition of a prayer, spoken in mantra-like rounds. Variations involve breath, movements, prayer beads, and other tools of the contemplative life.

Growing out of the practices of fourth century Cappodocian monks, *hesychasm* culminated in the fourteenth century writings within the Eastern Orthodox Church.

Archbishop Gregory Palamas and his fellow hesychists were greatly influenced by the first century theology of St. Symeon. Particularly instructive was his *Three Methods of Attention and Prayer,* which Matus refers to as "a manual of Christian yoga because it teaches the contemplative to link the invocation of the name of Jesus with awareness of heart and breath rhythms."

The message of St. Symeon, radical at the time and perhaps even today, is that direct experience with God—unmediated by priests, denominational mandates or theological hierarchy—is available to us all. Advocating for a practice based on a simple verse like the Jesus prayer, he was creating an accessible path to theosis—union with God—based on an oral tradition of repetitive prayer passed down from Desert Mothers and Fathers of the fifth century.

Avoiding the dogmatism he so carefully avoided in his own theology and spiritual life, Symeon did not advocate for one right way to practice hesychastic prayer. Even using the Jesus prayer was a choice, not a requirement. The Eastern Orthodox tradition considered other prayers just as effective in developing a personal practice of hesychastic prayer. The Prayer of St. Ioannikios the Great was one such alternative prayer, popularized in the seventh and eighth centuries: "My hope is the Father, my refuge is the Son, my shelter is the Holy Ghost, O Holy Trinity, Glory to You." The common denominator, of course, is the invocation of Jesus through the words of the prayer. The Jesus prayer may be said fully, "Lord Jesus Christ, Son of God, have mercy on me, a sinner," or partially, "Lord Jesus Christ have mercy on me." In its most basic form, it can simply be the word "Jesus" whispered by expectant lips.

Symeon garnered numerous yogic comparisons, due in large part, to his incorporation of breath-work into the practice. Like *pranayama* in yoga, the breath grounds the spiritual content of the prayer in the physical realm, forcing the mind and body to work together. Again providing room for personal application of the process, there are several ways to tether oneself to the breath. These include saying the entire prayer on an inhale followed by an exhaling of the whole thing. Alternately, the call to God (Lord Jesus Christ, Son of God) can be inhaled, while the cry for mercy (have mercy on me, a sinner) is exhaled. Yet another variation is to retain and hold the breath for a few seconds between the inhaled and exhaled portions.

Symeon's work proved to be a launching point for others within the Eastern Orthodox monastic tradition who continued to delineate the process of holistic prayer, providing a helpful paradigm for Christians seeking to enrich their prayer life beyond the comfortable realm of the intellect. This evolution continues to this day, as evidenced by the twentieth century work of Father Archimandrite Ilie Cleopa who established nine levels of prayer leading to theosis, or union, as:

- The prayer of the lips
- The prayer of the mouth
- The prayer of the tongue
- The prayer of the voice
- The prayer of the mind
- The prayer of the heart
- The active prayer
- The all-seeing prayer
- The contemplative prayer

Rather than literally prescriptive in nature, the list strikes me a bit like the reminders that lead us into *savasana* at the end of class. We are told to relax our eyebrows, our temples, our tongues. Our solar plexus, our kneecaps and our arches. Suddenly, through simple attention to these oft-forgotten regions, we are relaxed. We arrive at *savasana*. Likewise, if we are conscious of praying with lips, mouth, tongue, mind and heart, incorporating active prayer to an all-seeing God with a contemplative, receptive approach, we arrive at God's feet. In both cases, as if through some process not completely of our own doing.

A meaningful comparison of yoga and *hesychasm* shows that it is, indeed, not the physical grounding—the posturing, breathing and chanting—that we must examine, but the interior work being done. Matus articulates this, saying:

> Physical procedures are but the skin of yoga; its sinews and skeleton are mental exercises that lead to the transformation of consciousness. But the soul of yoga is a vision of light which is one, pure, undivided, and beyond all movement and change. How similar or dissimilar yoga and hesychasm really are can be seen only by comparing the highest spiritual experience proper to each.

From where I sit—whether on my mat or in a pew—I think Matus' "vision of light which is one, pure, undivided, and beyond all change" fits Jesus pretty well. I can attest that both Jesus, as the embodiment of God, and yoga, as my tethering practice, serve to point me daily to the great I Am. The one beyond naming, who I choose to call Sophia.

LECTIO DIVINA: DIVINE READING

Another practice which sprung from this still pool of *hesychasm* was *lectio divina*, literally translated as divine reading. The hesychastic Jesus prayer provided a physical link to the divine using voice and breath, while *lectio divina* was a means of connecting with God through the actual text of scripture. The scriptural basis made it an easy jumping off point for Christians already in the practice of memorizing, quoting and steeping themselves in God's word. Formalized by St. Benedict and Pope Gregory I in the fourth century, *lectio divina* was inspired by the Apostle Paul who said, "The word is near you, on your lips and in your heart" (Romans 10:8).

During this pre-Gutenburg era when monks often spent years of their lives copying scripture onto parchment, the sublime practice of *lectio divina* provided a very personal doorway into the text that could otherwise lose its meaning through the sheer roteness of monastic experience. Twentieth century French Benedictine scholar and author Jean Leclercq, speculates that it was the clandestine scribbling of favored passages, selected during the transcription process and tucked away for private meditation by monks during the Dark Ages that led to the advent of *lectio divina*. Unlike other contemplative practices that began in the Eastern Church and spread westward, *lectio divina* is rooted in Roman Catholic monasticism, making it somewhat more palatable and familiar to Westerners looking for disciplines to enrich their spiritual life.

The four phases of *lectio divina* are reading, meditation, prayer, and contemplation. During the first phase, the selected passage is read aloud, slowly and deliberately. Phase two begins when we stumble upon a word or phrase that seems intended for us that day. The meditation is our perusal of that word or phrase—a gentle tumbling of the words through the filter of our unique experience and worldview. In phase three, we take the tumbled words, softened and familiar now, and bring them to God in prayer and meditation. Finally, in phase four, we sit and listen, in a state that is paradoxically expectant and free of expectations, waiting for God to distill the wisdom we've gleaned down to its very essence. We make the words part of our breath and our blood, an internalized eucharist.

Regularly scheduled intervals for *lectio divina* in both personal and communal settings are a hallmark of St. Benedict's enduring contribution—the Benedictine Rule—which has become Western Christianity's leading guide for monastic living. While at first glance the rigidity of Benedictine's Rule seems at odds with the fluidity and ruminative nature of *lectio divina*, both serve the express purpose of removing the practitioner from the chaos of the exterior world, allowing the interior experience to move to the forefront.

BENEDICTINE RHYTHM: INTENTIONAL LIVING

Benedict formulated his now-famous rule during a self-imposed period of exile, a literal enactment of the archetypal quest for spiritual indwelling.

Thomas Moore, in his introduction to *The Rule of St. Benedict*, humanizes the saint's monastic journey. He provides us with the picture of youthful discontent and disconnection which led Benedict—and can lead us—to a state of equilibrium:

> Fifteen hundred years ago, a young man studying in Rome became disgruntled with the paganism he saw there and decided to live in solitude in a cave some distance outside the city. In that decision Benedict enacted a fantasy that has influenced the hearts of men and women— the idea of making a life apart from the crowd, in a style at odds with the norm.

Influenced by the same Cappodocian monks who embraced and formalized the spiritual concept of hesychasm several hundred years earlier, Benedict used the hesychastic solitude of his years in the cave to formulate ways in which monks could live communally, while retaining the element of withdrawal that sustained him during his formative period of seclusion.

Perhaps due to the increasingly frenetic pace of life, this type of simple, intentional living has struck the imagination of the mainstream. Through Julia Roberts' depiction of a spiritual pilgrim in the blockbuster movie based on Elizabeth Gilbert's *Eat, Pray, Love,* we can observe how ashram living in India resembles life in a Benedictine monastery. Both revolve around a balancing of prayer, work, leisure, and rest, a schedule which is surprisingly adaptable to modern non-monastic living as an individual or within a family unit. In his pocket-sized guide to living, *Always We Begin Again: The Benedictine Way of Living*, John McQuiston II reinterprets the Rule of St. Benedict, providing us lay people with a way to imbue every nook and cranny of our daily experience with sacredness, that in our minds is all-too-often reserved for clergy.

While the actual rule has plenty of obscure instructions clearly meant for monastics—*Chapter 31: Qualifications of a Monastery Cellarer* (the monk who manages the monastery's food supply), for example—the rule, overall, is a kind of spiritual predecessor to modern self-help books that endeavor to teach us how to use our time wisely. In the case of Benedict's Rule, it is not the hyper-productive type of multi-tasking advice we're likely to encounter in twenty-first century America, but rather a kinder, gentler approach to time management. A way to create a daily flow that keeps us grounded. McQuiston sums up his impetus to using the rule's principles in his own life, saying, "Time is our ultimate currency; we must be careful how we spend it."

His Benedictine-influenced weekday schedule includes seven stopping points that correspond, roughly, with the seven worship services inter-spersed throughout a monk's daily monastic duties. This modern interpre-tation of the rhythm interjects spaces to check in with our spiritual selves in the midst of the productivity that defines our work days. Because the rule was written to accommodate a self-sustaining, hard-working commu-nity, its modern adaptation is doable, even for the biggest type A's among us. Many of the stopping points are only a minute in length; however, despite their brevity, they are sacred moments, crucial to maintaining the balance St. Benedict envisioned.

During the peak busyness of our day, three such one-minute breaks are scheduled to allow us to say a quiet thanksgiving—10:30-10:31, 11:59-12:00, and 2:30-2:31. I waste much more time than that each day flitting around Twitter. The simple act of setting time aside to intentionally give thanks can be life-altering, a bit like a living gratitude journal.

Through careful appropriation of time, moderation—the bedrock of Benedict's rule—emerges as a construct for shaping human life to divine purpose. Through guidelines, instructions, and rules, it creates a frame-work that imposes moderation and restraint from the outside in.

How we fill the assigned blocks of time is as important as the act of assigning them. If, for example, we decide a healthy rhythm includes a modicum of downtime prior to bed, we will reap very different results by choosing meditation over media consumption as our way to unwind. Culturally, we have become incredibly desensitized to media—the sen-sory stimulation, the speed with which information is transmitted, and the prevalence of violence—believing that we're not affected by it. Both sleep problems and sleep-inducing medications seem to be on the rise, however, and I can't help think that filling our heads with images more conducive to a peaceful night's sleep would help. A brief meditation pe-riod before bed sets the tone for a restful night, just as one in the morning sets the tone for the day to come.

These Benedictine-esque practices are clearly aligned with the yogic *yama* of *bramacharya* (sensual restraint & moderation) and *ahimsa* (non-violence), linking the practice of yoga back to early monastacism in practical, doable ways.

CHANTING, MANTRAS & PSALMODY: GIVING VOICE TO OUR FAITH

One of the most confusing and misunderstood areas of yoga is the practice of chanting, whether it's a simple "ohm" to open class, or a *"shanti, shanti, shanti"* (peace, peace, peace) before parting. Yogis traditionally chant in Sanskrit, a beautiful, melodious language that seems to have been created from the purest vibrations in God's repertoire. Just try doing a full-bodied "Oooohhhhhmmmm" right from your belly, and you'll see what I mean.

Jesus' native tongue, Aramaic, shares the melodic, chantability of Sanskrit. Both languages developed during the same period (around 1,000 BCE) in the same broad geographic area of the Middle East. While I have yet to encounter a yoga teacher who chants in Aramaic, I did happen upon a breath-taking rendition of the Lord's Prayer chantingly sung in Aramaic by Australian-based world music duo Indiajiva on their album *Sacred Ragas*. If you had any doubt about the chant-worthiness of Christian prayers this will put them to rest.

It was my affinity for this distinctly Eastern *apophatic* (mistery-filled) experience—the feeling behind words chanted in a language my intellect could not decipher—that fueled my desire to incorporate mantra and chanting into my yoga practice and my faith. Feeling divinely inspired, I signed up to spend an evening meditating and chanting with Srivatsa Ramaswami, a highly respected chant master in India, also the author of several popular yoga books in the US, including *The Complete Book of Vinyasa Yoga* and *Yoga Beneath the Surface*.

I was particularly intrigued by the latter book because of its premise, which is basically the publication of an ongoing email dialog between an Indian guru and an American yogi. I wondered if it would address some of the stumbling blocks I'd come across in integrating this ancient Indian practice into my modern American (and Christian) life. And indeed, it did.

Presented in an accessible question-and-answer format, the conversation within the book covers practical issues such as the role of breath in an *asana* practice, then it veers into unexpected depths, tackling prob- ing philosophical issues, like whether yoga can lead you to happiness. Of course, as with any of the really important issues in life, others' ideas and opinions can only serve as guideposts God has placed in our lives to help us find our own way. Ultimately, the path is ours to choose.

So, as I immersed myself in mantra yoga with Ramaswami and a dozen or so eclectic practitioners, I felt a bit like I was sitting in on a church service of an unfamiliar religion. While we weren't speaking in tongues exactly, the language and the way it rolled off my tongue were distinctly foreign, yet comforting at the same time.

I grew up in South Texas, a land devoid of Jewish influence, but the chant- ing reminded me of an Indian version of Bat Mitzvah scenes I'd seen on TV and in movies. Beautiful melodious words pouring forth, their sacredness clear, but their exact meaning eluding me, *apophatic* in its mystery.

We chanted a wonderfully universal mantra about energy and peace an auspicious 108 times. I surprised myself by resisting the temptation to count, instead relying on Ramaswami to tell us when we were finished. I didn't have a sense of time passing as we chanted. When we were done and I was amazed I had stuck with it through the 108 repetitions, he asked us to silently chant the same mantra for ten minutes. Again, I had no aware- ness of time passing—no glimpses at my watch, no thoughts of how many minutes we had left. I did, however, find my thoughts wandering much more often during the silent chanting than in the previous vocal round.

For a beginner like me, it was much easier to keep my thoughts moored to the tangible action of voicing my mantra than to the silence that al- lowed distractions to creep in and disrupt the sacred space I was creating in myself through the mantra.

Psalmody—literally translated as singing the psalms—is the closest approximation we have to yogic chanting in our mainstream Western Christian tradition. The practice transferred seamlessly from the Jewish psalters and was transmitted strictly orally—*viva voce*—until they were committed to paper using a rudimentary form of musical notation un- der the watchful eye of Pope Gregory, for who they were named, around 600. By the time they were codified and standardized as Gregorian chant,

St. Benedict—born sixty years before Pope Gregory—had already popularized their use among monastics by including the practice in his rule, which was quickly becoming the standard structure for European communal faith communities.

The Gregorian chant of the Middle Ages—ethereally voicing the mystery of the contemplative soul—became the keystone of monastic liturgy, performed seven times each day, including a particularly arduous 3 a.m. offering. These very same chants—recorded at a little-known Spanish Benedictine monastery and titled simply, *Chant*—became an unexpected pop culture phenomenon in the late 1990s, bringing the very idea of Christian chanting to the attention of many people for the first time.

But being introduced to their beauty did not inspire a resurgence of Gregorian chanting among the masses. Why? Well, first of all, many of us can't sing. While they were technically chanting, those monks clearly used some serious musical ability to paint the most haunting of melodies with their voices. No one was offering Gregorian Chanting 101. Those inclined to chant, it seemed, rather liked the mind-numbing vibrational repetition found in Eastern chanting. Avoiding complicated lyrics and intricate melodies, yogis typically engage in chanting to escape the head and retreat into the spirit. The pendulum among yogis and other contemplatives had swung decidedly toward the *apophatic* (mysterious) and away from the *kataphatic* (linguistically or otherwise defined) spiritual work. With chanting, this means less formal, both in lyrics and melody, to allow for a personal spiritual experience to emerge from the process. It is analogous to a repeating a simple one-word mantra rather than a long rote prayer.

I saw no reason I couldn't take all that I'd learned and experienced and apply it in a Christian context. Still, I yearned for someone to guide me into the realm of Christian chanting. I wanted affirmation from within my own faith tradition that I'd stumbled upon a profoundly transformative practice. I wanted my voice to join a symphony of other seekers calling out to God. Repeating ourselves, not so God could understand us, but so we could understand God.

In Benedict's rule, we find a glimpse of this mystical musical potential. Within its inherently rigorous structure, these gentle words encourage us to pursue our authentic voice, "Let us consider how we ought to behave in the presence of God and his angels, and let us stand to sing the psalms in such a way that our minds are in harmony with our voices." This is what I feel when I'm chanting in my yoga practice—that my mind is in harmony with my body. The chanting becomes an audible manifestation of this yoking. The sound of wisdom, Sophia speaking. Could it really be that this same principle—of sacred vibrations carried on modulated, mindful breath—has been at work in my faith tradition all along?

When we take the words of the Bible at face value—as flat, one-dimensional messengers of God's living word to us—we overlook the true power of chanting the psalms. The same thing happens when we fail to recognize the transformation that occurs within us through the process of chanting and instead turn it into a performance for God. The same God who already knows every hair on our heads—knows every curse word we've ever muttered under our breath, every evil eye we've ever shot at someone—and loves us anyway. Without an *apophatic,* wisdom-seeking intention, our chanting can become just another of our misguided attempts to earn the divine favor that's ours for the taking. We can easily forget that there are no strings attached, nor choral coups required for communion with Sophia.

So if we're not performing our chants to earn God's love, what defines their transformative nature? Four distinct elements turn psalmody into a form of Christian yoga which Bourgeault described as "a highly precise system of inner alchemy...that produces definite changes in the subtle energetic structure of their being." The spiritual fruits of chanting—whether the words are Christian, Hindu, Jewish or Buddhist—are real. This is not imagination, nor is it heresy.

Breath... The *prana*—the vital life embodied in our breath—fuels every chanting practice. As important as the breath is in an *asana* practice, it is absolutely essential for chanting, serving as the vehicle upon which the words traverse the divide between our interior and exterior worlds. Beyond the physical transformation brought about by the oxygenation of the body's cells, lies the crux of the metamorphosis: that breath and spirit are one. In most languages, the same word is used for both. Chanting can only penetrate into the realm of the sacred if carried on the breath.

Tone... This is the result of the breath doing its deep, sacred work—the sounds pushed up and out from our center. This center, in terms of our physical acoustics, is the diaphragm. If our utterances don't emanate from our center, we are presenting the world with a facade, with something other than—less than—our true selves.

Intentionality... The *logos*—the words themselves—have always been primary in Christian chanting. Rather than losing ourselves in the words, we are meant to find ourselves. We do this by paying attention to the way in which our utterances echo back and speak to us. Like a *lectio divina* set to music. Within a vibrational framework, we intone carefully chosen words with the intention of unifying ourselves with God through the *logos*. This brings us full-circle, our chanting becoming one vehicle through which the true meaning of yoga—the yoking of ourselves to God—is realized.

Community... While it is possible—sometimes even desirable—to chant in solitude, there is a reason we typically do it communally. Just as singing a solo is different from singing in a choir—the former is likely to engage the ego, the latter a spirit of cooperation—chanting takes on a richness when our voice melds with others, adapting and harmonizing to chords rising up from those around us. That first "ohm" of any yoga class can be pretty pitiful. The room veritably vibrates with dissonance as unfamiliar voices bump up against one another. It seems like a bit of yogic alchemy to me that these same voices somehow align themselves over the course of the class and emerge in perfect harmony for the concluding "ohm."

An interesting variation on chanting within the Christian faith is to pray the psalms, rather than chant them. While this is often done audibly, its intention is more akin to that of the *lectio divina* than to true psalmody, where the tone and musical elements play a key role. I was first introduced to this practice by Jerry Webber, Director of the Center of Christian Spirituality, in his seasonal devotionals, *Sometimes an Unknown Path* and *Fingerprints on Every Moment*—both subtitled *40 Psalm Prayers in Contemplative Voice*. Originally written to walk one through the liturgical seasons of Lent or Advent, these books revealed a new way of praying for me, an intriguing interaction with words that made them come alive and made me feel they could awaken parts of my soul too.

Starting by praying the psalms in a methodical, orderly manner just as Benedict did some 1,500 years ago, Webber committed to praying ten psalms a day, covering the entire body of 150 psalms in fifteen days. Eventually, he extended his practice to the creation of his own psalm prayers that captured the essence of these sometimes baffling Old Testament verses that spoke passionately of violence, revenge, and other unsavory urges we all try to repress—as if it were possible to hide them from God.

In a poignant example of the transformative power of this practice, he relates his experience in the psalm-prayer that came out of reading and meditating on Psalm 137, an incomprehensibly violent expression which is, understandably, often avoided by lay people and clergy alike. The psalm reads:

> *Remember the day of Jerusalem, O Lord,*
> *against the people of Edom,*
> *who said, "Down with it! down with it!*
> *even to the ground!"*

> *O Daughter of Babylon, doomed to Destruction,*
> *happy the one who pays you back*
> *for what you have done to us!*

> *Happy shall he be who takes your little ones,*
> *and dashes them against the rock!*

How do you meditate fruitfully upon a text that culminates in the dashing of infants upon rocks? Webber explains his approach to the inherent violence and avarice of this verse, taking the humble position that even these most abhorrent feelings are alive in him—alive in all of us. Rather than leaving us to ruminate on words that may evoke depressing feelings, psalm-prayer writing helps us take the words in, mold them within our being as they course through our veins, beat within our heart, and finally take root in the soul. What emerges from that process is his own psalm prayer which gives voice to *ahimsa*—non-violence, our first yogic *yama*.

> *Don't let everything You've built in me*
> *go for naught.*
> *Don't let it be leveled by my own arrogance,*

or by the cruel intentions of others.
I'm tempted to yell and scream,
"Get them before they get me!"
I'm tempted to lay off all my troubles on those who surround me
while I'm away from Home.
But I got myself into this place.
I thought I knew best.
I turned my back on You.
I set out on my own course.
I don't need retribution toward my enemies
—I seem to be my own worst enemy—
I need a generous spirit toward my flattering self
and toward them.
Don't do violence to anyone.
but bring each of us into our true Home
in you.

In a typical yoga class you are going to encounter Sanskrit chants, not Benedictine psalmody or cathartic pslam-prayers. Though these vocal forms share the same underlying structure and form, you may find yourself stumbling over the Sanskrit, wondering about the meaning of the words you're chanting. So, how do you handle unknown words uttered in a language considered dead outside of sacred settings (much like Latin for Christianity)? Part of the process is simply switching from our Western *kataphatic* (known) default mode into *apophatic* (unknown) mode where we can experience without intellectual understanding. Chanting's wisdom comes from the breath, tone, intention and community, not from the lyrics.

Many oft-chanted Sanskrit terms, including *shanti* (joy) and *pratibah* (light), serve as universal invocations of the divine. The popular Gayatri mantra exemplifies Sanskrit chanting that bridges the gap between yogis' varied religious beliefs:

Oh, God I (we) meditate on your divine light. Bestow your blessings on us so that my (our) intellect may be enlightened, so that I (we) may rise higher and higher to the highest consciousness. Enable me (us) to meditate, to be successful in all affairs of life, and to realize God (Truth).

This mantra is reflective of the God realization I experience in Sophia who embodies divine truth in a way that's unencumbered by definition, unhindered by theology. Other, less literal chants, particularly those featuring Hindu Gods or Goddesses, require a more metaphorical interpretation. A perfect example of this kind of chant is *Sita Ram,* which reverberates with the repeated invocation of the names of the divine couple Sita and Ram as a call to unification of our feminine and masculine sides to bring about wholeness. The concept is not contradictory to other faiths, though the actual names may be stumbling blocks if taken literally. When seen as symbols of the duality that exists in all of us, Sita and Ram become melodious signposts of truth and wisdom, rather than a God and Goddess pulling us away from the truth of our own faith tradition. This embracing of metaphor serves as a point of connectivity between faith and yoga, creating a spiritual experience that's bigger than any one religion.

When we approach our yoga practice—including its vocal portions—from a wisdom perspective, embracing the *apophatic* way of unknowing, we paradoxically begin to know in a way that's deeper and more profound than we did before. Sophia emerges on our exhaled breath, carried on words spoken in the language of the heart, not the mind.

Your comfort level with Sanskrit chanting from the Hindu tradition is between you and God. I have journeyed through this quandary for the almost twenty years I've been practicing, and, for the most part, I am comfortable with my *apophatic* approach to the tongue the yogis use to communicate their faith. It is beautiful. Lyrical. Vibrational. And it soothes my soul. That I know. Just as I don't stop going to church because a sermon rubs me the wrong way, I don't stop going to yoga class when I come across a chant or mantra that is not my cup of tea.

You may encounter a specific chant invoking Hindu theology that takes you beyond your own comfort zone. An example of such a chant, for me, is the classic Invocation of Patanjali which choruses the Sanskrit words for:

I pray at the lotus feet of the supreme guru who teaches the good knowledge, showing the way to knowing the self-awakening great happiness; who is the doctor of the jungle, able to remove the poison of the ignorance of conditioned existence.

To Patanjali, an incarnation of Adisesa, white in color with 1000 radiant heads, human in form below the shoulders holding a sword, a wheel of fire, and a conch, to him, I prostrate.

This chant, designed to honor the yogic sage Patanjali, may be used by a teacher of any class that adheres to Patanjali's eight limbs of yoga. I have found, however, that many mainstream teachers shy away from it, perhaps realizing that it may stir up consternation in students. In my own discernment, I am not comfortable praying at the feet of a deity-like guru, even a symbolic one, when I can't draw at some sort of analogy to my own belief system. So, when I encounter a passage or prayer like this, I silently invoke the wisdom of Sophia, praying that all who are present will be touched by a God who is here and with them, even if they call that God by a different name than I do.

Jesus' propensity to go where others didn't and to visit places not sanctioned by the church is my inspiration to take my faith with me into yoga class. Many yoga practitioners have been wounded by religion. By bringing our own imperfect embodiment of Jesus' teachings into these spaces in a quiet and contemplative way, without an agenda to convert or proselytize, you may be giving others their very first glimpse at a Jesus unencumbered by formal interpretations. Chanting alongside others can sometimes do more to build spiritual connections than preaching to them.

The ultimate work of chanting, psalmody, mantras, and psalm-prayers is to give voice to spiritual longings we may not recognize. To pray the words our own tongues do not know. We borrow and recite. Internalize and absorb. Until one day, our voice is indistinguishable from God's. They have become one. We become the authors of our own psalm-prayers, the utterers of mantras that vibrate through our beings, binding us to something bigger and grander than our fumbling selves. We embody yoga by speaking its sacred language.

The literal language you choose matters little—Sanskrit, Latin, Aramaic, or plain old English will do nicely. God understands them all. The intention-filled context within which you place your words is what transforms them from mere syllables to God-speak. There are no rules. No one gets to decree which holy intonation is best for you. My advice? Try them on for size. Play with them. Don't be afraid of sounding silly. And let me know if you happen upon a new variation or approach that draws you closer to God. For someone who can't carry a tune, I am insanely interested in this particular mind-body connection that rides on our breath directly to our soul.

MUDRAS & MALAS: FINGERING OUR FAITH

"We are physical creatures, and concrete reinforcements of habits of meditation, prayer and gratefulness will assist us in the work." – John McQuiston II (Always We Begin Again)

What could be more of a concrete reinforcement than one we can hold in our hand or form with our fingers? Just as our voice can tether us to the here and now of meditation, accoutrements of faith can prop up our flagging attention when we need it most. Whether born of what we already are (*mudras*) or an adornment representing what we want to be (*mala*), these sacred hand gestures and prayer beads are used in virtually every faith on the planet.

Too often dismissed as Eastern by Christians, the viability of these two very tangible contemplative traditions has been all but lost on modern day spiritual seekers outside the Buddhist and Hindu worlds. As with every practice we've looked at, these two yogic tools have surprisingly strong roots in Christianity, as well as other faith traditions.

Mudras

Because they require nothing but your own hands, *mudras* are a most portable and economic practice. While yogis have traditionally used *mudras* in conjunction with meditation in seated postures such as lotus, half-lotus, or *samasthiti* (simple seated pose), no mat and, indeed, no particular posture is required to invoke the power of a *mudra*.

Like *asanas* for the hands, *mudras* are simple gestures that focus or direct energy during a yoga practice, prayer, or meditation. Three *mudras* which overlap into Christianity via the art and tradition of Byzantine and Greek churches are the *prithvi, pran,* and *anjali mudras. Privthvi mudra,* in which the thumb and ring finger are joined, is said to provide stability and cure weaknesses of the mind and body. *Pran mudra* is formed by connecting the pinky and ring finger with the thumb. The resulting symbol is said to increase vitality and protect the body from disease, particularly when combined with the breath (*prana*) for which it was named. Finally, there is the universal *anjali mudra*—hands pressed together at the heart's center, the heart chakra. *Anjali,* literally translated as "offering," "a gesture of reverence," "benediction," or "salutation," is derived from "*anj,*" meaning "to honor or celebrate."

Though inexorably linked to the Indian traditions of yoga, Hinduism and Buddhism, *mudras* crop up more often than you might imagine in the art and images of other faiths, particularly that of Eastern Christianity. Byzantine-style paintings of Christ, the Virgin Mary, angels and saints—hands poised mid-*mudra*—attest to the hidden role of *mudras* within Christianity.

Mudras—like so many contemplative Christian practices—began in the East and flowed westward, mixing and mingling with neighboring religions while passing through fingers of different faiths. Staring at Jesus, hand poised in a perfect *prithvi mudra,* I feel like my worlds have connected along with his fingertips, my Christian beliefs mystically melded to my yoga practice by his hands.

Apparently, I am not the only one to intuit the spiritual power of this delicate hand gesture. Even today, Greek Orthodox priests place their hands in this *mudra*—sometimes referred to as the Sign of Benediction—as they make the sign of the cross while speaking a blessing. In ancient frescoes, Christ is also depicted in *pran mudra,* a particularly apropos choice for Jesus the healer, and a wonderful way for us mere mortals to embody his healing energy and to align our intention with his.

The ubiquitous *anjali mudra* is a prayerful posturing adopted by practitioners of all religious backgrounds. While the term "*mudra*" is usually only applied in Eastern contexts, the essence of the posture is shared across geographic and religious boundaries each time hands come together in prayer. Often used as a welcoming or parting gesture in yoga classes, it is more than a superficial greeting.

Anjali *mudra* is a physical expression of yoga's inherent yoking. By pressing our palms together, we emulate the unifying of ourself with the divine, passing this intention on to others with a slight bowing of the head. Not coincidentally, our hands typically assume *anjali mudra* when our lips utter *"namaste"* at the end of class. They are two ways of saying the same thing. One is for the ear, the other for the eye.

Refreshing in their universality, *mudras* silently communicate the heart of yoga, reminding me of St. Francis of Assisi's famous quote, "Preach the Gospel at all times and when necessary use words." Without using a word, *mudras* capture the spirit of both yoga and Christianity, enabling us to share it with others.

Malas (Prayer Beads)

Prayer beads share this universality, yet serve a more personal, less outwardly expressive, function. Rather than gesturing to another, they tether us to ourselves, keeping us present, each bead a moment that we experience, not intellectually, but tactilely. Passing beads through our fingers, we relieve our overburdened minds of their duty, shifting away from our hyper-intellectualized existence. As the secular name for prayer beads— worry beads—suggests, the kneading of the beads somehow takes our worries from us.

Variations abound under faith-specific monikers—*misbaha, tasbhi,* and *subha* in Islam; the Greek *komboloi*; *japamala* used in meditation by Hindus and Buddhists; rosaries and knotted prayer ropes for Christians. The word *bead* itself is derived from the Anglo-Saxon word *bede,* which means prayer, likely an etymological derivative of the Sanskrit word *bodhi,* which refers to self-realization or enlightenment. Beads, it seems, were destined to be tools of prayer.

This spiritual application is not lost on modern-day creators of these beautiful strands that could easily be mistaken for a yogic fashion statement. Diana Charabin, founder of Tiny Devotions, surmises their appeal saying, *"Mala* beads remind us that life is a prayer." This profound summation led me to interview her about the myriad of ways people use *mala* beads in their spiritual journeys.

In true yogic fashion, she focuses on the unitive rather than the divisive aspects of the *mala,* saying, "The commonality amongst all of these different beads is a tangible object which the wearer or user can actively use for prayer work, stress relief and cultivating intention." *Malas* are traditionally used in several ways—most commonly as a mnemonic to keep count of prayers or mantras (Christianity and Hinduism), and as a means of ticking off the mental conditions or sinful desires that one must overcome to reach enlightenment or nirvana (Buddhism).

While the particulars of a prayer bead practice vary among faith traditions, their ability to provide a touchstone for divine communion remains consistent. In fact, it is almost certain that prayer beads were introduced to Christianity via another faith. Some suppose that the Desert Mothers and Fathers adopted the beads as a result of encounters with Muslims or Buddhists along trade routes about a thousand years ago. Others see Christianity's rosary as an evolution of the Hebrew Psaltar of David that would have been practiced by Jews who became the first Christians.

While acknowledging the universality of their application, Charabin isn't naive enough to think that everyone has the instant comfort level and knowledge base needed to integrate *mala* beads into their spiritual life. She admits, "*Mala* beads or prayer beads are soaked with contradiction and confusion. Many guidelines and rules have been set up by different groups and cultures of how and why to use them. My take on it—and what I have found from my experience—is that their power lies in allowing the individual to apply their own meaning and their own set of rules on how they can use them in their daily life."

Even today, *mala* beads are often created following the Hindu tradition of stringing 108 *rudraksha* seeds to form the base of the necklace. *Rudraksha* seeds are popular because they are known in Indian culture for their protective and sacred qualities, though *malas* of wood, semiprecious stones and other natural materials abound. A hundred and eight of them because of the auspiciousness of the number in both religious and secular circles.

Like *mala* beads themselves, the number 108 has significance in many realms, both spiritual and scientific. Whether nature, sacred text, or metaphysics is your language of choice, you will find a correlation with this auspicious number.

So, why is 108 so great? Astronomically, the distance between the earth and sun is 108 times the diameter of the sun; the diameter of the sun is 108 times the diameter of the earth and the distance between the earth and moon is 108 times the diameter of the moon. The number is theologically significant to Christians, Jews, and Buddhists. The 108th verse of the Bible symbolizes yin-yang unity in Genesis 5:2, which says, "They were created female and male, given a blessing and named 'humankind' on the day they were created." In Tibetan Buddhists' belief system, 108 sins must be overcome in order to attain nirvana. In literary terms, Homer's Odyssey includes 108 suitors coveting Odysseus' wife Penelope; while anthropologically, the diameter of Stonehenge, perhaps the world's most renowned prehistoric monument, measures 108 feet. In *Ayurveda* (Sanskrit for "knowledge for long life")—ancient India's system of medicine—there are 108 pressure points in the body where consciousness and flesh intersect to give life to the living being, and 108 chakras or centers of spiritual energy in the human body.

Despite an adherence to traditional Hindu *mala*-making, modern mala wearers use their malas in a myriad of spiritual practices. Charabin elaborates,

"While *mala* beads are traditionally used for *japa* meditation—reciting Sanskrit and/or sacred transcendental sounds along the beads to purify their body, mind and soul—as the spread of *mala* beads grows, the shift in mantras has also expanded. Westerners unfamiliar with Sanskrit may now recite positive affirmations such as 'I am strong' or simply the word 'love' along the beads to change their vibration and set their intention for the day."

With this Westernization comes the inevitable effusiveness of our culture, expanding the scope of the *mala* beyond the personal and into the public sphere. Like charm bracelets encircling our wrists with glittery remembrances of our hobbies and loves, *malas* now beam out our intention to those around us, sometimes giving us a needed reminder in the process.

The *mala* serves as an outward sign of an inward desire to align with the principles of peace, unity, and love by ceasing a negative behavior or or initiating a positive one. According to Charabin, "A *mala* is a subtle energetic and physical reminder to live life to its fullest, stay present and focus on an area that needs cultivating." Some mala makers use semiprecious stones chosen to enhance specific intentions as the *mala's meru*—a larger bead, stone or knot marking one round of mantra or prayer.

Writer and vinyasa yoga teacher Insiya Rasiwala-Finn describes her experience wearing such a *mala* during pregnancy, aptly identifying it as an extension of her yoga practice:

> "Whether you believe in the spirituality of *malas* or enjoy them purely for their *sringaar* (decorative beauty), there is something both substantive and grounding about wearing a *mala*. For me, I have a little growing being deep in my belly and the thought of having a smooth yet irregular turquoise stone, (signifying communication, healing and balance) resting at my *hara*, or energy centre, the spot right where my baby lays, is comforting as I navigate my busy days. It feels like a protective, guiding amulet. I've come to think of wearing a *mala* to be an extension of my physical yoga asana practice, the door through which so many of us enter to go further. There's so much more available, but only if we want to go there. Wearing a *mala* can be a perfect entry point."

CENTERING PRAYER: CHRISTIAN MEDITATION

Malas are, indeed, a perfect entry point for those with a natural bent toward Eastern spirituality who are looking to expand their yoga practice beyond the physical realm. It is centering prayer, however, that is likely to be the first yogic-like encounter modern-day Christians have within their faith tradition.

Where Eastern Orthodox theologians and spiritual seekers left off, Western contemplatives picked up in the late 1970s with the advent of centering prayer. Influenced by contemporaries like Thomas Merton, monks at Massachusetts' Saint Joseph's Abbey—led by Abbot Thomas Keating—took the ninth level of prayer, designated as contemplative in Roman Orthodoxy, and brought it to life. To Westerners hungry for an intentional practice in which to experience the God of their faith tradition, this new way of praying was like having the words they had read and heard all their lives set to music—glorious, heart-wrenching, coming home kind of music.

Tremors had shaken our cultural foundation, creating fault lines in the religious status quo and receptivity among Christian spiritual seekers. Centering prayer was not the only form of Christian meditation to arise from the newly created chasms. In West London's Ealing Abbey, Benedictine monk John Main was beginning to teach his own form of Christian meditation. More akin to the type of mantra recitation that lends itself to *mala* beads, Main's method is said to be more focused on attention, while Keating's was more about intention.

The overarching quest in centering prayer—sometimes called contemplative prayer—is to rest in God's presence. To be and not do. Centering prayer is the yin to the yang of mantra and *mala*-based meditation which give voice to our prayers and put our fingers to work, counting and tracking our spiritual progress in rounds. In contrast, centering prayer leads us into stillness, ushering in silence, knowing that when we are silent, God ceases to be.

As Solomon wisely reminds us from the pages of scripture, "What has been before will continue to be, what has been done before will continue to be done—there's nothing new under the sun!" (Ecclesiastes 1:9). Centering prayer did not rise up out of the abyss in post-modern America, riding on the coattails of peace-loving hippies. It stems directly from *hesychasm*, a concept we have already traced back to the Desert Mothers and Fathers, and to Jesus before them.

Centering prayer is inspired most directly by the *apophatic* views first documented by Pseudo-Dionysius in the fifth and sixth centuries (*via negativa* or negative way) which focuses not on what we know about God, but on what we don't. Evoking the mystery of a pure entity, formless and unknowable in the realm of mental conception, centering prayer is a practice born out of this theology perhaps best articulated by an anonymous Christian mystic in medieval text, *The Cloud of Unknowing*:

> "For [God] can well be loved, but he cannot be thought. By love [God] can be grasped and held, but by thought, neither grasped nor held. And therefore, though it may be good at times to think specifically

of the kindness and excellence of God, and though this may be a light and a part of contemplation, all the same, in the work of contemplation itself, it must be cast down and covered with a cloud of forgetting. And you must step above it stoutly but deftly, with a devout and delightful stirring of love, and struggle to pierce that darkness above you; and beat on that thick cloud of unknowing with a sharp dart of longing love, and do not give up, whatever happens."

Like yoga and the meditative techniques associated with it, centering prayer mines the soul, revealing the mystery of what lies within, exposing it without seeking to define it. Sophia's wisdom—sacred yet formless—fills the resulting pits and pocks. Sometimes we walk away with precious stones, sometimes protective metals, and sometimes we're empty-handed. But never empty-hearted.

Because of its gentle nature, we hold loosely to an intention during centering prayer, rather than drilling it into our psyches with repetitious mantras, choosing a simple word that addresses (God, Sophia, Abba, Jesus, Mary, etc.) or expresses (love, peace, mercy, light, etc.) the divine.

We should hold the conventional practices of centering prayer—how long to practice and how to sit—as loosely as we hold our sacred word during our meditation. Indeed, all the practices we have looked at are just that—ways to practice communion with God. They were conceived by men and women on spiritual quests similar to our own, to light an inwardly spiraling path that leads to divine wisdom, Sophia.

While the term "centering prayer" is of modern origin, its essence has been living in the quiet, still spaces within Christian contemplatives since Jesus walked the earth himself, directing his followers in their spiritual lives, saying: "But when you pray, go to your room, shut the door, and pray to God who is in that secret place, and your Abba God—who sees all that is done in secret—will repay you" (Matthew 6:16).

Exactly how you will accomplish this shift from you to God is up to you, but the contemplative tradition offers guidelines that can serve as a roadmap of sorts as you chart your own course. On my own journey, I modify, combine, and tailor many practices listed to help me find my unique connection to God. In one sitting, for example, I may use *asana,* breathing, centering prayer, candle gazing, and a host of other tools to tether me to God. To find my center for that day. My practice might include reading scripture or other inspirational texts. It may involve writing or chanting. I may be called to movement or stillness. Your own practice will reflect your relationship to God at that point in time. Listen and God will guide you. Don't let others impose their rules onto your spiritual life.

As I continue learning who I am and who I'm not, it becomes easier to avoid the pitfall of comparing my insides to others' outsides. There is much nourishment to be found in the spiritual truths of others, as long as we use them to reflect upon, rather than to dictate, our own experience. I can still remember reading Sue Monk Kidd's brave and honest memoir, *Dance of the Dissident Daughter*, years ago and feeling that someone finally understood the longings of my heart that I was afraid to express. Her words both captured my heart and set it free. Thomas Merton's gentle prose and poetry have been another of my spiritual guides. While these two very different individuals share a connection to the feminine divine, I'm sure they both arrived at her feet by circuitous routes. And each path was just as it should have been.

More than a decade before his influence helped launch the centering prayer movement, Merton wrote an ode to the feminine divine of his experience titled simply, *Hagia Sophia*. I find it telling because the feminine face of God is not easily found in mainstream Christian denominations. She is almost always discovered while we are roaming the terrain of the soul in quiet contemplation. Her name isn't proclaimed from pulpits, and there are few signs pointing to her. We have to discover her ourselves as Merton describes in his 1963 *Hagia Sophia*:

There is in all things an inexhaustible sweetness and purity,
a silence that is a fount of action and joy.
It rises up in wordless gentleness and flows out to me
from the unseen roots of all created being,
welcoming me tenderly,
saluting me with indescribable humility.
This is at once my own being, my own nature,
and the Gift of my Creator's Thought and Art within me,

speaking as Hagia Sophia,
speaking as my sister, Wisdom.

While Merton, Keating, and other Christian contemplatives are adept at expressing the divine in a myriad of subtle voices—often evocative of the feminine and the natural world, they are deeply and irrevocably committed to Jesus as the embodiment of God sent here to earth for us.

Experiential faith practices may seem different from Jesus as we're used to encountering him in mainstream religion. Rather than a character in the story of God who we relate to alternately as a miraculous baby, crucified king or risen savior, he becomes a companion on a journey—transformed from an outer arbiter of our faith to an inner source of wisdom, leading us to Sophia. Seeking the mystery rather than knowledge of God broadens our theology to include a *sophiological* approach alongside the *soteriological* theology of the Western church. When we put on this cloak of mysticism, we begin to see wisdom everywhere. God suddenly turns up in the most unexpected places—in the words of a friend from a different faith background, the smell of soup on a cold winter night, or in the quiet of *savasana*. Attempting to sum up my own zig zag road to sacred wisdom, I could say that I subscribe to Buddhist philosophy (detachment, awareness, etc.), practice yoga (all eight limbs), and put my faith in Jesus who illuminates and embodies the perfect grace of Sophia.

Contextualizing a specific faith within a larger worldview is inherently difficult. Catholicism, which is often seen as backward to social progressives, has taken an astoundingly progressive stance, affirming the role of philosophy and reason in religion in recent decades. In his 1998 Papal Encyclical, "Faith and Reason," Pope John Paul II supports the exploration of self consciousness as a legitimate spiritual path, saying:

> In both East and West, we may trace a journey which has led humanity down the centuries to meet and engage truth more and more deeply. It is a journey which has unfolded—as it must—within the horizon of personal self-consciousness: the more human beings know reality and the world, the more they know themselves in their uniqueness, with the question of the meaning of things and of their very existence

becoming ever more pressing. This is why all that is the object of our knowledge becomes a part of our life. The admonition 'Know yourself' was carved on the temple portal at Delphi, as testimony to a basic truth to be adopted as a minimal norm by those who seek to set themselves apart from the rest of creation as 'human beings', that is, as those who 'know themselves.'

And what did Jesus practice in his own life? Jesus the yogi. Is it really that far fetched? These two verses tell me that it's not:

> Jesus insisted that the disciples get into the boat and precede him to the other side. Having sent the crowds away, he went up to the mountain by himself to pray, remaining there alone as night fell...At about three in the morning, Jesus came walking toward them on the lake (Matthew 14:22-25).
>
> After sunset, as evening drew on, they brought to Jesus all who were ill and possessed by demons. Everyone in the town crowded around the door. Jesus healed many who were sick with diseases, and cast out many demons...Rising early the next morning, Jesus went off to a lonely place in the desert and prayed there (Mark 1:32-35).

The Jewish term for prayer, *tefillah*, does not denote the beseeching we often associate with prayer, rather it was a way of life, a means of communing—not communicating—with God. The spiritual aim of *tefillah* is to discern what is within oneself, to help us see who we are in God's eyes. Prayer permeated the days of Jews in Jesus' day. While Paul's admonition to pray without ceasing (1 Thessalonians 5:17) seems an impossibly high standard today, it was, indeed, the expectation among Jesus and his contemporaries. To Jesus, however, merely praying incessantly was not enough. Sitting quietly, reflectively, alone in God's presence was so important to Jesus that he used this secluded form of prayer both to prepare for a miracle (in Matthew) and to recover from performing one (in Mark).

Sitting on a mat, arms and legs folded in quiet contemplation would be very much in character for the Jesus we learn about in the Bible. The one who steals away for time to meditate in lonely spots and on mountaintops.

The one who defends Mary's own quiet contemplation as she sits and washes his feet, soaking in his words and his very presence. This story of two sisters, from Luke 10:38-42, tells us that simply being with God can be more important than doing godly deeds, as it juxtaposes the ways in which Mary and Martha interacted with Jesus. Martha scurries about busy preparing a meal for Jesus and his traveling companions who have come to visit the sisters and their brother Lazarus. Mary, conversely, sits at Jesus' feet listening in a way that is typical of a student-teacher relationship, oblivious to all the last-minute details consuming Martha. Unable to bear the injustice any longer, Martha storms over and demands that Jesus tell Mary to help her in her righteous work. Jesus surprises everyone saying that it is Mary who has chosen to focus on the most important work of all.

Does that mean that Jesus didn't appreciate Martha's hard work—or the work we undertake in his name? No, of course not, but it does show his desire for us to balance the inner work with the action he calls us to in our lives.

Mary was listening to Jesus, not only to his words, but to his demeanor, to his every move. She was in tune to him. Martha, while busy with God's work, was not nearly as aware of Jesus' presence. So often in my life I find myself in Martha's shoes—trying to do the right thing while not taking the time to really listen to Jesus.

By adopting an apophatic stance, we learn it's alright to just sit and listen, ceasing to fear the unknown. A bent toward a sophiological understanding of Christ opens us to wisdom-seeking, altering our prayer life. Our prayers begin to overflow their banks and infiltrate our lives. We move toward a place where simply by living, we are praying without ceasing.

I have learned this skill—this way of attentive listening—from my yoga practice more than any from any other teacher. On my mat, I feel wisdom. I test its truth and learn to embody it. When my *asana* practice is over and I roll up my mat, the truth stays with me. Yoga has become my *tefillah*, my unceasing prayer.

CHAPTER 4

Lessons from the mat

STANDING TALL, SOPHIA RISING INTO THE BODY
THAT IS HOME TO MY SOUL
BENDING FORWARD, BOWING TO THE DIVINE.
ARCHING BACKWARD, OPENING MY HEART
TO WHAT IS.

TWISTING DEEPLY, WRINGING MY VERY CORE,
UNSEEN EMOTIONS, THOUGHTS AND FEELINGS
CAREFULLY HIDDEN
COME UNBIDDEN INTO THE LIGHT.

BREATHING THEM OUT WITH EACH EXHALATION,
BREATHING IN GENTLE MERCY AND
UNCONDITIONAL LOVE
FILLING ME WITH THE KNOWLEDGE
THAT I AM RIGHT WHERE I SHOULD BE
AT THIS MOMENT.

MOVING INTENTIONALLY, EMBODYING A
SACRED GRACE
THAT COMES FROM A RESERVOIR DEEP WITHIN.
MEDITATING ON THE WATERS OF THAT
MYSTERIOUS PLACE
NOTICING THE RIPPLES ON ITS SURFACE.

I OPEN MY EYES,
SEE NO WATER
BUT FEEL ITS UNDULATIONS ALL THE SAME.

CLAIMING THAT VIBRATION,
ITS FREQUENCY UNIQUE TO ME,
I ROLL UP MY MAT.

GRATEFUL FOR A PRACTICE
THAT TRANSCENDS THIS SPACE,
THIS TIME, THIS BODY.

NAMASTE.

I wrote this poem to explore the intersection of my faith and yoga, trying to express how they come together in my practice. My most profound yogic lessons are those that I am able to take with me when I leave my mat. There is something about learning holistically—that is with my body, mind, and spirit—that just makes it stick. I can read something and know it in my head. I can hear something and it may penetrate all the way to my heart. I may even remember these things and share them with others. But there is something about learning by doing that takes me beyond knowing and into the deeper waters of believing.

I'll tell you about my friend's experience. In the midst of a huge life transition as she prepared to return to work after staying at home with her two boys for a number of years, she was nervous, unsure of the abilities and skills she hadn't exercised in quite some time. She was scared that her talents had atrophied and afraid she wasn't ready for all that would be required of her on an upcoming week-long international trip, her first since re-entering the professional world. She needed courage. She didn't need to read about it or even to hear someone tell her she had it. She needed to experience it for herself.

She went to yoga class and focused on something other than her fear. The teacher was working on backbends that day, using the wall as a support to encourage the students to trust, as they bent unseeingly backward, that the wall would be there for them. It was more of a mental than a physical hurdle for most of the students, and many hesitated, not willing to throw caution to the wind and fling themselves backward. My friend took a deep breath, and back she went. The teacher, not one to lavish praise on students, noted how brave she was for doing that. And suddenly, she felt brave. She didn't intellectually think she was brave, she felt courage travel through her body and right into her soul. She was ready for her trip in a way she hadn't been before that class.

God has a way of working through yoga to teach lessons that we desperately need to learn. As you might expect if you've had some experience with God's brand of instruction, the lessons don't often come in those glory moments when we've just nailed that posture that's been kicking our butt for months. They come with the herniated disc (humility) or the pulled groin (patience) or when we're trying desperately not to think about our to-do list while lying in *savasana* (being in the moment). They come, basically, when we least expect them. But, this I promise you—if you get on that mat and work your yoga, the lessons will come. Here is how I've experienced God teaching through yoga.

HUMILITY

We all have areas of our lives that we can become prideful about if we don't consciously cultivate humility. Cultivating sounds like such a painless, methodical effort. I wish that I'd had the foresight to proactively cultivate humility surrounding my yoga practice. But I was too busy raising kids, running my business, and trying to get something reasonably healthy on our dinner table each night to consciously cultivate anything. I was in a constant state of reaction. I knew that yoga would counteract this reactive state, but I simply wasn't coming at it with the right attitude. I was carrying my competitive attitude right onto my mat.

So, instead of cultivating humility, I was hit with it over the head—or maybe whacked in the back would be closer to the truth. I was very proud of my yoga poses—of my flexibility, which I didn't have much to do with anyway. One Saturday I was holding my two-year-old on my hip and bending down to pick up firewood. When I straightened up, I felt it. And it wasn't good. It wasn't subtle. And it certainly wasn't painless. I barely managed to avoid dropping my son along with the firewood. Whatever this was I didn't have time for it. I needed to fix it. Now.

I had a herniated disk, which, among other things, required me to refrain from forward bending for three months. It was just not possible for me to look like a hot shot yogi when everyone else was bending over with their hands on the floor and I had my hands on my upper thighs, giving my injured back the mere ten degrees of flexibility it would provide without causing me to spasm in pain. As those three months drug on, and I began to get used to being the least flexible person in the class, I began to gradually shed that pride I had clung to for so long. Because of my physical limitation, I had to make a choice. I could either continue my practice with its modifications and a dose of humility or I could cling to my ego and quit, cocooning myself away until I could emerge and begin aiming for perfection. I chose to try humility and began doing my yoga for

126

me, for where I was that day, and not for the sake of doing it better than the person next to me.

PATIENCE

Because neither yoga nor life in general are linear experiences (as much as we'd sometimes like them to be), many of the lessons I've learned are intertwined. For example, while learning humility through my back injury, I was also learning patience. Patience in that only God knew when my herniated disc would repair itself. The doctors could make an educated guess, and I could squirm with anticipation or try to force the healing process, though neither of these worked very well for me. I had to live *apophatically*, embracing the unknowing. People think I must be patient to do yoga when, in fact, I do yoga to become more patient. Some say that they can't do yoga because they can't sit still. Well, that is precisely why they should do yoga. We don't water a flower *when* it blooms, we water it *so* it will bloom. I don't wait for God to bestow the gift of patience on me before unrolling my yoga mat. Instead, I unroll it and say a prayer for patience—just for that hour. Then I do my part to cultivate patience—that is, do my yoga. There's that word cultivate again. I hate it, and I love it. It is not a revolutionary word. It is not an exciting word. It is a word that denotes doing the next right thing and waiting for the seeds of your labor to sprout—perhaps many months from now. But I find that what I practice on my mat does, eventually, make it off the mat and into the rest of my life. Yoga teaches traits holistically, so that the same patience I used with my back injury, found its way into dealings with my children, husband, friends and clients.

LIVING IN THE MOMENT

Yoga lures me back to the present moment. Every time I try to focus on a specific muscular adjustment instead of my grocery list. Each time I watch my thoughts float away and bring my awareness back to my breath. Each time I remind myself that it doesn't matter how cute my yoga teacher looks in her coordinating outfit, while I'm in my sweats. Once again, the lessons intertwine, reminding me not to covet my neighbor's stuff and shift the focus from external to internal.

The art of living in the moment does not belong only to yogis. The Benedictine monks who pioneered the monastic life in southern Italy in the sixth century beautifully embodied this quality. The sect was led by Benedict of Nursia, a Roman noble who, despite being canonized by the Catholic Church in 1220, never set out to found a religious order. He had the same longing many of us have today—a longing to live life in a simpler, more meaningful and purposeful way. When he left Rome and headed into the countryside at age twenty, he knew that he believed in God and in Jesus as his savior, but he also knew that church as it was done in Rome wasn't working for him. Sound familiar?

Like so many people I know, I found myself on that same quest, looking for an authentic way to live out the life that Christ had called me to live. I knew that the church experiences I had found didn't embody this calling, but I didn't know what did. Today—as in centuries past—people like Saint Benedict are still questioning the status quo and finding new ways to live and worship in community. Yoga was part of that rethinking for me. It slowed me down enough to hear God's voice to which I had become deaf after so many years of tuning it out. I perceived such a huge discrepancy between what I knew about God and what I saw in my encounters with organized religion. I couldn't reconcile it, so I stopped trying.

Once yoga had me tuning in again, God led me to a beautiful community of believers where my faith was able to blossom. I was attracted to that community because I sensed that it was filled with people authentically seeking God's will in a way that seems very much in line with many of the ideals Saint Benedict put forward in his famous Benedictine Rule. In one of our church's very first small groups, we studied McQuiston's translation of the Benedictine Rule. When we entered the doors of the old church sanctuary, we left behind the worries of work and small children. Of mortgages and bills. We ate soup—slowly and quietly. If you want to have a contemplative dinner together, I highly recommend soup. Soup does not lend itself to shortcuts. Its very nature requires a slow lifting of the spoon—over and over again. It slides down your throat in a way that allows you to feel it making its way into your body, its warmth spreading calm that brings you into the moment—whether you want to be there or not. While the heart of our group's purpose was finding ways to live out ancient monkish precepts in a modern world, the soup was the vehicle that readied us for the contemplative mind our task required.

GRATITUDE

Words of gratitude can have such power in my life—when I just remember to use them. At times when I have consistently kept a gratitude journal, I (and my family) have noticed a marked difference in my demeanor. It is absolutely true that the states of mind that steal our serenity—anger, resentment and self-pity—cannot co-exist with gratitude.

When yoga is practiced as a lifestyle, rather than an exercise regime, its implications extend way past the mat. Recently, I was lying on a blanket in my backyard, soaking up that mixture of warm sun and cool air that makes Houston simply intoxicating in the early spring. I took off my glasses and laid back looking at spring swimming before my eyes in a cacophony of colors and realized that people with perfect vision never get to look at the world in this mystical kaleidoscopic way. I was suddenly profoundly grateful for something lacking in my life. I was grateful for the beauty I was finding in the imperfect vision God had blessed me with. I never imagined I'd find myself filled with gratitude for eyesight that would render me legally blind without correction. It was the observation skills I'd learned in my yoga practice that helped me make this unlikely connection to gratitude, and to embrace the ambiguous aura as a glimpse into the mystery that Sophia continues to reveal to me.

I can't see the big "E" on the eye chart. When I first got my glasses in second grade, I was amazed that trees had individual leaves (they weren't just the big green blobs I drew with my crayons) and that stop signs actually said STOP (they weren't just drops of red planted at intersections). I resented being the only one of four sisters in my family who couldn't function without glasses, a resentment that peaked during my teenage years. Now it's just a part of who I am. But, grateful? No, my poor eyesight has never quite inspired that before.

I have been grateful for the fact that it is correctable and have reveled in its seemingly miraculous return each morning when I put on my glasses. This kind of gratitude flows naturally upon the return of something we have missed.

So, deprivation that leads us to gratitude is not a new concept for me. But gratitude *for* the deprivation—for that moment only and not some final destination or ultimate "correction" of the deficiency—is one I discovered that spring day on the blanket because of yogic seeds that had been planted and cultivated over years of practice, both on and off the mat.

THOU SHALT NOT COVET THY NEIGHBOR'S _____

For me, it's thou shalt not covet thy neighbor's perfect backbend. For you, it might be the never-ending headstand or the unbelievably flexible hips situated on the mat next to you. It doesn't matter. Even in the distinctly noncompetitive world of yoga, I have found myself comparing and, at least in my own mind, competing. The absurdity of realizing that I am on a yoga mat, and still wishing I had what the person next to me does that finally compelled me to change the old tape in my head that kept telling me I have to *do* more to *be* more.

Making the *yama* of non-covetousness (*aparigraha*) part of an *asana* practice is key to integrating this lesson, but for me, progress started when I was able to embrace *ahimsa*, the very first *yama* of non-violence. When I was able to put my well-being ahead of my quest for perfectionism, I began to let go of my yoga envy and start practicing the *niyama* of contentment (*santosha*). On the mat, that meant not pushing past the point where I felt compression in my lower back during a backbend—even if it meant I had a less spectacular backbend—because I was committed to a practice that nourishes, not harms, my spine. I had to let go of a lot of ego in the process, acknowledging the sudden headaches that would come on if I went into extreme backbends, and admitting that the pain was God's way of telling me to back off. After years of practicing backbends in a kinder, gentler way (with props if necessary), I can't say that I have an envious backbend, but I can say that I don't spend much time envying others' backbends. Instead, I go into my own body and focus on the cues—usually some variation of "don't poke your tailbone out"—that I've learned through self-study (*svadhyaya*) keep me out of pain and in my practice.

It also helps to remember that the yogi I may be envying is a *vision* of perfection, not perfection. I have no way of knowing what's going on inside another person's pose. By making other practitioners (and all those other perfect mirages we encounter daily) so in our mind, we create un-realistic expectations for ourselves. I have a favorite ritual for reminding myself that those visions of perfection dancing in my head aren't real. I sit down with a cup of hot tea, and I drink it from a beautiful, misshapen cup a dear friend of mine made. When she made it, it was so misshapen that my friend's fellow ceramicists assumed she would throw it away. My friend saw something beautiful in it though. She fired it with inspirational messages on both sides. One side says, "I am imperfect but worthwhile." The other says, "A mistake a day keeps perfection at bay."

Tangible touchpoints, whether an *asana*-based attitude adjustment or a hand-held mantra like my misshapen mug, are ways of accessing faith te-nets in everyday life. The ideal of non-covetousness found in nearly every faith tradition comes alive when placed in a yogic context.

THY WILL, NOT MINE

When we let go of our will in a yoga pose, we open up a space in our practice for God's will. This is where the magic really starts to happen. This is when you move deeper into a pose than you've ever gone before. It is a physical manifestation—a lesson right there on your mat—that teaches you the power of letting go and letting God. It shows us that God's will is always better for us than ours.

So what if you let go and you don't feel the magic? Sound familiar? How many times in our lives have we turned something over to God and then immediately doubted because what we wanted to happen didn't? Your pose may not look any better. Heck, it may not even feel any better yet, but if you are breathing through it and keeping your mind on it, you are making progress. And, after all, God is all about progress, not perfection.

In my own practice, it's become clear that God's will is for me to be-come stronger. I need strength to stabilize my poses and to avoid hurting myself. My will relies, instead, on flexibility and avoids the work it takes to cultivate strength. I take the short-cut. The path of least resistance is just too tempting for many of us to resist, both on and off our mats.

Yoga *asanas* have become a laboratory where I experiment as I learn to discern my will from God's—physically trying things my way then noticing the difference when I decide to follow the voice calling me to something deeper and truer. Simpler or subtler. The voice of Sophia. This discernment is the wisdom we seek through faith, and yoga becomes a practical route to that wisdom.

SUBMISSION & SURRENDER

I have always had an issue with the word submission. The resistance stems from the fact that the church seems to have spent an inordinate amount of time and energy advocating for the submission of women to men. In an effort to impose this one-sided concept on often unwilling subjects, the focus on true spiritual submission—or surrender, has been lost.

Whether we're surrendering our will to God or yielding to each other as we merge two lives in a committed relationship, there is a grappling with and ungripping of long-held beliefs that must happen. Initially, this engages muscles, bones and joints, using the physical body to pierce our awareness. Through a yoga practice, we can learn to see our bodies, and in turn our spirits, as they really are, rather than how we wish they could be. Once we are holding firmly onto our truth (*satya*), we are better able to decide what aspects of our lives need to be submitted or surrendered.

Eckhart Tolle describes the process beautifully in his book, *The Power of Now*. He talks of surrender as an acceptance of what is—a process that leads us to drop our inner resistance, or constant state of discontent—that creates negativity. My yoga teacher, Selise Stewart, claims that no growth in our practices ever happens without surrender. As is often the case, she is talking about yoga, but the lessons she is teaching go way beyond the mat.

In a yoga practice, you must surrender to the aching muscle or to the tight hamstring in order to move beyond them and go deeper into the pose. As in childbirth, the real pain comes not from the process, but from the resistance. When I gave birth to my children, at the times I was truly able to relax into my contractions, I experienced relief. The pain did not engulf me and I could work with it for a greater good. In labor, as in yoga, it is not necessary to do this without help. Props are yogic tools for accessing the deeper experience of a pose while working within physical limits.

In yoga *asanas*, blocks, belts, and bolsters are there to offer support when you need it. Surrendering resistance does not mean giving up the right of self-advocacy. To the contrary, it means knowing yourself and your needs well enough to reach for the right tool to help your body to drop its resistance to the reality of a pose. I've found when I have practiced this on a physical level, I am much more adept at doing it emotionally. The tools look different, but the results are the same.

Yoga is not about internalizing others' answers, but about finding your own. As a yoga practitioner, it is your work to define your own boundaries—to discover when you need help, when you need to push through and when you need to back off. An experienced yoga teacher will give you pertinent information when you need it—like never, ever push past pain in your knee joint—but will let you experiment within safe parameters, empowering you to take responsibility for your own practice. We can have much the same experience in our spiritual lives if we can learn to perceive and rely upon the sacred wisdom being imparted to us all the time. The mat is a wonderful place to begin that journey.

BALANCE

Everything about yoga embodies balance—from the *yin* and *yang* so often used symbolically within a yogic context to the actual physical balance required in many of the *asanas*. Balance, in conjunction with breath, is the core element of any type of yoga *asana* work. For every move in yoga, there is a simultaneous countermove designed to create balance in that pose. Once the balance is achieved, the stillness follows. And then, finally, in the stillness, the mind begins to quiet itself.

Initially, we tackle the large, obvious adjustments as we seek equipoise in our bodies. Some are an effort to achieve symmetry between the left and right, or front and back sides of our physical frame. Some—like chest opening—are meant to counterbalance the excesses of our Western culture. Without vigilance to taking the shoulders back and allowing the heart center to move forward, we end up stooped from the large blocks of time many of us spend working on computers, driving, and in other stances that work with gravity to bow our shoulders.

To give an example of a more subtle balancing action, in standing poses where the legs are together, teachers often cue us to roll the tops of our thighs in toward one another. This is a small, but important, movement because it gives stability to our base. However, if left unchecked—or un-balanced—this necessary adjustment results in the tailbone sticking out. The rolling in of the thighs must be balanced with a gentle pulling down of the musculature that covers the buttocks. The willful, goal-oriented version of this balancing movement would be tucking the tailbone. Focusing on moving the the gluteal muscles forward is more difficult, more subtle, but, ultimately, more balancing.

Another example of balance in action occurs when the shoulder blades are pulled down and back to open the chest. This tends to cause the ribs to jut out. They must be brought back in alignment with the rest of the torso in order to balance the action of the shoulders and to maintain a truly erect spine. This happens by lifting the back of the rib cage. Talk about counterintuitive! I never even realize there was a back side to my rib cage until I began working on this particular balancing action, which is key to my practice.

Most obviously, balance is cultivated in yoga class by learning to main-tain equilibrium—not toppling over—in a pose that requires such action. These may be one-legged poses, the most basic of which is *vrksasana* or tree pose. While, at first, most students will try to will themselves to stay upright, eventually they will learn the subtle, non-physical keys that will bring them the balance they are seeking. It is not the focus on the trem-bling foot that will bring the balance. What we focus on expands, or—in this case—trembles even more!

What will finally bring the balance is the stilling of the mind, which can come through any of a number of meditative techniques. Simple things like focusing on your breath, holding your eyes on one unmoving spot in front of you (a *drishti*), or visualizing your standing leg rooted in the ground with a continuous flow of energy going up the front and down the back can help. Notice that even visualizations require balance to be successful. Watching the energy flow up but not down (or vice versa) will not bring about balance.

BEING WHERE YOU ARE

Yoga is such a great teacher of this lesson. Each time we do a yoga *asana*, we are challenged to stay with a pose, to stay in *our* yoga—whatever that may look like on that particular day. Doing this means not taking short cuts to make ourselves look good. It's doing the hard work, sticking with the discomfort (not pain), and learning to work in a deeper and healthier way.

In tree pose, it may mean keeping the bent leg on the ground instead of hoisting it up against the knee where it's going to cause joint issues down the road. Once you can get it to stay up on your inner thigh, then you work there. Until then, your work may not look glamorous, but it is your yoga for that day.

It is tempting to find shortcuts in a pose—like sticking out the ribs or tailbone to make a pose easier. When those in class do this, our yoga teacher says we're doing our neighbor's yoga, not ours. And she's right. We may be forcing our bodies into a position that resembles the ideal pose, but, in truth, we are emulating, imitating life rather than living it.

Off the mat, there are many temptations to take actions that make us look good, but miss the point. Who cares if you have a mcmansion but your kids never see you? Or if you are going into debt to live in the "right" neighborhood or belong to the "right" club? These are examples of doing your neighbor's yoga. It is an easy trap to fall into, but I've found that a yoga practice can provide a way to counter cultural tendencies that go against our personal grains. By grounding ourselves in a physical practice that speaks to us in spiritual ways, we are able to hear the voice of wisdom—Sophia—and we are empowered to act on it. To be who we are no matter where we find ourselves.

Ultimately—and thankfully—God created each of us as unique and wonderful beings. Our challenge is to keep our mind in our own head and keep our focus on ourselves. Not in a self-centered way, but in a way that allows us to live out our truths, not somebody else's. Only then can we begin to contribute to the world in an authentic and meaningful way. Only then are we doing our own yoga.

ACCEPTANCE

After doing *trikonasana* (triangle pose) for almost fifteen years, I was given a cue in yoga class that totally changed the way I saw the pose. I realized that the version I had been doing all these years was not the real pose after all. It was a version I had created that looked technically correct, but lacked the deeper awareness and alignment that this new cue brought into my pose.

My first reaction to this enlightenment was not thankfulness for a new understanding, but dismay and indignation that after fifteen years, I couldn't even do *trikonasana* right. Now my hips were facing the floor when I had worked so hard for years to square them to the front. When I voiced these thoughts to my teacher, she responded, "It looks like you have some work to do. That's the beauty of yoga. Wouldn't it be boring if we learned the pose perfectly and then never had to work on it again?"

With a sigh that was the beginning of acceptance, I brought myself back to the present and started working—painfully, slowly—toward restoring my hip alignment within this new awareness. It was so much like the work I do off that mat that I just had to laugh. I am rarely happy when God decides to teach me a difficult lesson. I am almost always thankful for the lesson after it is learned, though. Someday I will be happy that I am doing triangle pose in a way that is good for my body rather than doing one that just looks good on the outside. And those off-the-mat lessons God teaches me through Sophia's whispers? I'll be grateful for those too.

WHEREVER YOU GO, THERE YOU ARE

When we recognize ourselves as unique creations of a loving God and begin to live our lives in accordance with this belief, we must also acknowledge those habits that rear their heads again and again, disrupting the peace God intended for us. If left unchecked, we will continue to experience the same problems over and over again because we are not aware of what's causing them.

We can practice awareness of habits in the physical realm of yoga practice, and that enlightenment will go more deeply into our mental habits as well. When we cultivate this awareness and begin to detect our own physical and mental idiosyncrasies, we then realize that they are not isolated to one specific situation—or, in the case of yoga, to one pose. For example, if a practitioner collapses her arches while standing in *tadasana* (mountain pose), she will then go into a balancing pose and collapse the arches there too. The collapsed arches have become part of her stance and approach to practice, and it will follow her into the next pose, unless she stops and deals with it.

Like bigger emotional issue that we face in life, the simple act of bringing our awareness to these habits is the beginning of the end for them. Once we bring something out into the light, it loses its power over us. A collapsed arch no longer equates to a constant state of irritation for you in standing poses. It becomes just what it is—a physical glitch that you have identified and can work on, ignore, or accept. The choice is yours.

LET IT FLOW

After Hurricane Ike's landfall on the Houston/Galveston coast, my family and I weathered the storm—and its 100+-mile-per-hour winds that whipped through our heavily wooded yard—huddled together in the family room, which we had decided was the least likely spot to have a tree come through the roof. As it turns out, we were right. The trees did fall, but on other parts of our house—one falling on, but not puncturing the roof, and the other coming through the roof and breaking water pipes in our attic. We spent the two weeks moving from hotel to hotel, trying to keep life for us and our two children as normal as possible.

I have a tendency to minimize my feelings, and because I was staying in nice hotels, eating good food and, generally, remaining free from much of the trauma of the storm, I didn't let myself grieve—didn't let myself feel what I was feeling. Others had it so much worse that I didn't think I deserved to be sad. But denying feelings does not make them go away. They stay around and fester, and they will come to the surface eventually as an emotional blow-up like rage or depression or even manifest physically.

With the help of a particularly cathartic yoga class, I was able to let them flow. After almost two weeks of running on adrenaline and holding life together without any of the familiar comforts of hearth and home, I just let it all go. Big tears ran down my face during *savasana*. I didn't judge myself for them or try to justify them, I just accepted that they were there, running down my face, and that was where I was at that moment.

My yoga teacher noticed the little river flowing onto my mat. And she handled it beautifully, simply placing a small towel over my eyes, completing the cocoon of my internal focus. After class she said, "You really need to be back home, don't you?" She was right. But despite the fact that

I still didn't have my physical home back, just by letting myself "go there" emotionally, I felt I was coming home in an even more important way. As I have often experienced, God has a unique way of teaching me. We got power the next day.

THE LESSONS THAT KEEP ON GIVING

In yoga, as in life, lessons are not learned linearly and they are not learned only once. Three years after learning humility from my herniated disc, I found myself right back in the same place. Intellectually I know that the lessons learned on the mat are not one-time-shots, but I was still flabbergasted and angry to find myself back in the same pain.

Doing a yoga class with a new teacher, I pushed myself into a pose that just didn't make anatomical sense to me. The teacher was young and a dancer, so maybe it made sense for her. Because I was not as in-tune to the wisdom of Sophia as I later became, instead of doing my yoga, I chose to do my teacher's yoga. Instead of listening to Sophia telling me I should back off and stay with the first (not that impressive-looking) level of the pose, I plowed ahead, forcing myself into the pose. I just couldn't resist the challenge. More honestly, I couldn't resist the chance to show off.

As soon as that moment of glory had passed, and I was moving back into my down dog, I knew I had made a mistake. My lower back was screaming and tears were coming to my eyes. I have a tendency to look at the world in very black and white terms—things are either perfect or horrible—and I saw my current pain as a carbon copy of my past injury. I immediately fast-forwarded to physical therapy sessions, weeks of pain, and months of an extremely limited yoga practice. I started beating up on myself for going there—for doing that pose that wasn't in my best interest just to prove that I could. Who in the world was I trying to impress?

Mentally, I was taking my past and making it into my future. I was all over the place—moving back and forth in time and resting everywhere but the present. But perhaps I had made more progress than I realized. Suddenly, I was able to see this new pain was what it was—an experience in and of itself—not related in any way to my previous injury. When I realized this, I returned to the moment and finished my yoga class doing only what I knew wouldn't aggravate the injury. I sat back and wiggled my hips in child's pose whenever the class pose didn't work for me.

Once I was able to separate this new injury from my past one, and release some of the fear that I felt thinking about reliving that particular previous pain, I was able to see my current situation for what it was and for what it wasn't. It wasn't the debilitating injury of my past. As my beloved chiropractor said when she saw me the next day, "You're gonna live." And sure enough, just days later, the excruciating pain I had dreamed up and envisioned for myself was merely an annoyance, hardly registering as I went about my day.

Through this process I learned to let myself experience the lesson God is trying to teach me rather than trying to foresee the outcome before God has even gotten started working on me. This time, I just needed a gentle prod, a reminder to be grateful for the healthy body God has given me. I didn't need a major breaking down. I just needed to stop focusing on what was wrong with my body and start enjoying all that I can do with this body I've been blessed with. That may not look exactly the same at forty as it did at twenty-five, but that's OK.

The shift was definitely more inward than outward. I still work to fit in time in my day to nourish my physical self. What's changed is not the content of my life, but the intention that propels it. Instead of using self-criticism as my workout fuel, I am now running on gratitude. The results may be the same, but the journey is very, very different.

TAKING IT OFF THE MAT

Think of your yoga mat as a launching pad for life. In order for yoga to become a true tool for transformation, you must take what you learn off your mat and into your everyday life. Otherwise, your yoga practice is just a glorified form of exercise or an escape from the real work that is your life.

In yoga poses, we often make the most progress with the least effort—that is, with the least willful, goal-oriented type effort. You can't force your way into longer hamstrings or more open hips. If you do, you'll end up with an injury that will lead you straight into those lessons on humility and patience.

When you let go physically, heeding Sophia's wisdom, you can't help but stop coveting. When you let go—of your expectation of yourself, of

139

your image of yourself in the pose or what the other people in the class think of you—you are entering a yogic mindset. Until then, you are practicing, warming up for the real thing. Not that that's a bad thing. Everyone's timetable is different. It's not about how "good" you are at yoga. I think I spent a long time in rehearsal mode because, paradoxically, the poses came easily to me.

My mind wasn't nearly as nimble as my body. A teacher once had a class stop and look at one of my poses, saying they may never see one like this again. I was filled with pride that I now understand was misplaced. My interior yoga was out-of-whack for days.

It is an intentional cultivation of this interior yoga that is the crux of our practice. The benefits of yoga confined to a mat are very limited. We all know the feeling of hearing something that really resonates with us, some important truth we had forgotten, feeling really moved by it, and then promptly forgetting it. This often happens to me at retreats. I go. I am inspired. I am full of convictions and ideas I want to implement in my life, and excited about the new friendships I want to pursue when I return home. But then reality sets in, and because I don't make time to meditate on those truths, they are forgotten. Or I don't take any action toward keeping those new friendships going, and they wither on the vine. God always provides another opportunity for me to soak up truth and wisdom along with plenty of chances to act on them. But how much easier would it be if I didn't wait for an organized retreat to slow down and listen for Sophia's voice, putting her wisdom to work in my life daily? What if I created a mini-retreat for myself every time I stepped on my mat? Wouldn't that keep me in closer contact with God? Yes, it would. And it does when I remember to do it.

This conscious contact with God can only happen if I am creating a sacred space for it—making it a priority and giving it a spot on my calendar. It can so easily get edged out by the demands of life. As I learn to take the stillness cultivated on the yoga mat into everyday life, I am edging closer to a state of praying without ceasing. I am listening and responding to Sophia, and you can too.

When I make space in my life for yoga, it creates space within me, giving me a dependable touchpoint that I can go back to when things are spinning out of control. It may be just sitting on my mat and breathing before anyone else wakes up. It may be a down dog snatched between carpool and the grocery store, or a mantra recited before a trying situation. I don't know what it will look like for you, but you and God can figure that out.

Yoga leads me closer to belief and bolsters my faith when it wavers. The story of Charles Blondin illustrates the power of true belief, the kind of belief that can only come from doing.

The French tightrope walker wowed crowds in the summer of 1859 by traversing the gorge below Niagra Falls on a rope suspended 160 above raging waters. Being the first person ever to do so was not enough for the Great Blondin. Over the course of the summer, he invented and enacted a myriad of treacherous variations on the famed tightrope walk, all without the security of a safety harness. Each time he stepped onto the rope on the American side, the audience of up to 100,000 spectators held their collective breath, and when he set foot on Canadian soil, they cheered uproariously.

With the nonsensical antics of a Dr. Seuss character, he walked across the gorge on stilts, blindfolded, in a sack, even with a stove and chair in tow, sitting down mid-way across to cook and eat an omelette before finishing the feat. One day he crossed with a wheelbarrow filled with a hundred pounds of potatoes, or 350 pounds of cement, depending on which report you believe. The crowd went wild with applause following each exploit.

Blondin, emboldened by his success, turned to the crowd and asked if they thought he could push a man across in the wheelbarrow. "Yes! Yes! Yes!" they roared, chanting his name approvingly. Addressing one particularly enthusiastic fellow, Blondin queried, "Sir, do you think I could safely carry you across in the wheelbarrow?" Without hesitation, the man replied, "Yes, of course!" With a smile and a flourish, Blondin said, "Get in." The man refused.

This man clearly believed with his head that Blondin could carry him safely across, but that kind of knowledge doesn't always translate into action. He wasn't willing to live the belief that was firmly planted in his intellect. The beauty of learning by doing is that the action is built into the lesson. When I experience a truth on my yoga mat, I am much more likely to carry it with me than I am after reading a book or hearing a sermon on the topic. It becomes a part of me, another lesson learned through Sophia's infinite wisdom. So as I roll out my mat, and get to work, I hope you'll join me. It's not nearly as daunting as jumping into Blondin's wheelbarrow.

CONCLUSION
living with sophia

IN PROVERBS 8:27-31, SOPHIA CLEARLY TELLS US THAT
SHE WAS WITH GOD FROM THE BEGINNING OF
CREATION, SAYING:

> I WAS THERE WHEN THE ALMIGHTY CREATED THE HEAVENS,
> AND SET THE HORIZON JUST ABOVE,
> SET THE CLOUDS IN THE SKY,
> AND ESTABLISHED THE SPRINGS OF THE DEEP,
> GAVE THE SEAS THEIR BOUNDARIES
> AND SET THEIR LIMITS AT THE SHORELINE.
> WHEN THE FOUNDATION OF THE EARTH WAS LAID OUT,
> I WAS THE SKILLED ARTISAN STANDING NEXT
> TO THE ALMIGHTY.
> I WAS GOD'S DELIGHT DAY AFTER DAY,
> REJOICING IN THE WHOLE WORLD
> AND DELIGHTING IN HUMANKIND.

In the contemplative Christian tradition of *lectio divina,* we are asked to listen to a passage, not just with our ears, but with our hearts. We are asked to hear the one word or phrase that speaks to us and then to listen again, more deeply, to what God is speaking directly to us through the scripture. In this case, I hear "delight" so clearly. I know that God is giving me Sophia as a sort of spiritual playmate, a divine soulmate. I hear God saying that Sophia was here from the beginning and is here with me now. I don't have to understand exactly who Sophia is or how to define her. Really, can any aspect of God be truly divine if human definition can encompass it?

If contemplative wisdom could be condensed down to just one word, it would be this—listen. "Ausculta!" Benedict commands in the first word of his famed rule, reminding us to listen, deeply and reverently. Trying to explain this spiritual sense of hearing, David Steindl-Rast writes, "For just as the eye perceives light and the ear sound, the heart is the organ for meaning." I believe that the voice we hear when we follow our heart is Sophia's. The meaning we glean from it is her wisdom and becomes ours.

As I practice stillness through yoga and meditation, my mandate is to surrender to the mystery. It is continually revealed to me that I need to embrace Sophia, not as a religious icon, but as the face of God that lives in me. She is my Holy Spirit personified. Breathe her in; let her reveal to you the deep spiritual wisdom God is trying to impart. Yoga, in its fullest form, provides a structure that makes that possible.

Bibliography

Bell, Rob. *Love Wins: A Book About Heaven, Hell, and the Fate of Every Person Who Ever Lived.* San Francisco: HarperOne, 2011.

Bourgeault, Cynthia. *Chanting the Psalms.* Boston: Shambhala Publications (New Seeds), 2006.

Bourgeault, Cynthia. *The Wisdom Jesus.* Boston: Shambhala Publications, 2008.

Charabin, Diana (founder, Tiny Devotions). Interview via email, May 2011.

Christian Yoga Magazine, *Yogic Mudras in Christian Imagery.* http://christianyogamagazine.com/christian-yoga/yogic-mudras-in-christian-imagery/, 2009.

Christians Practicing Yoga, www.ChristiansPracticingYoga.com.

Christian Workers Magazine, Volume 16, *Have You Believed and Committed?* Chicago: Moody Bible Institute, 1915.

Coyle, Kevin. *Back to School, Back Outside: Create High Performing Students,* National Wildlife Federation, 2010.

Deignan, Kathleen. *Thomas Merton: A Book of Hours.* Nortre Dame, IN: Ave Maria Press (Sorin Books), 2007.

Frenz. Albrecht. *Yoga in Christianity.* Madras, India (now Chennai): The Christian Literature Society, 1986.

Gannon, Sharon and David Life. *Jivamukti Yoga.* New York: Ballantine Books, 2002.

Gates, Rolf and K. Kenison. *Mediations from the Mat.* New York: Anchor Books, 2002.

Gilbert, Elizabeth. *Eat, Pray, Love: One Woman's Search for Everything Across Italy, India and Indonesia.* New York: Penguin Books, 2007.

Idliby, Ranya, Oliver, Suzanne and Warner, Priscilla. *The Faith Club.* New York: Free Press, 2007.

Jacobs, A.J. *The Year of Living Biblically.* New York: Simon & Schuster, 2008.

Jones, Timothy Paul. *Praying like the Jew, Jesus: Recovering the Ancient Roots of New Testament Prayer.* Clarksville, MD: Messianic Jewish Publishers (Lederer Books), 2005.

Kadesky, Elizabeth. *First There Was a Mountain: A Yoga Romance.* New York: Little, Brown and Company, 2004.

Kidd, Sue Monk. *Dance of the Dissident Daughter.* New York: HarperOne, 1996.

Kushner, Lawrence. *Jewish Spirituality: A Brief Introduction for Christians.* Woodstock, VT: Jewish Lights Publishing, 2001.

McQuiston, John. *Always We Begin Again: The Benedictine Way of Living.* New York: Morehouse Publishing, 1996.

Matus, Thomas. *Yoga and the Jesus Prayer Tradition.* Mahwah, NJ: Paulist Press, 1984.

Mendel, Heather. *Dancing in the Footsteps of Eve: Retrieving the Healing Gift of the Sacred Feminine for the Human Family through Myth and Mysticism*. Winchester, UK: O Books, 2009.

Merton, Thomas. "Hagia Sophia," *The Collected Poems of Thomas Merton*. New York: New Directions Publishing, 1977.

Neyrey, Jerome. "The Idea of Purity in Mark's Gospel." Semeia 35 (1986):91-128.

Niequest, Shawna. *Cold Tangerines*. Grand Rapids, MI: Zondervan, 2007.

Paul, Russil. *Jesus in the Lotus: The Mystical Doorway Between Christianity and Yogic Spirituality*. Novato, CA: New World Library, 2007.

Puthenpura, Cherian. *Yoga Spirituality: A Christian Pastoral Understanding*. Bangalore, India: Camillian Publishing, 1997.

Ragel, Ron and Hansen, Vicki (Indiajiva). "Lord's Prayer" (Abwoon D'bashmaya), Sacred Ragas: http://www.youtube.com/user/indiajiva

Ramaswami, Srivatsa and Hurwitz, David. *Yoga Beneath the Surface: An American Student and His Indian Teacher Discuss Yoga Philosophy and Practice*. Boston: Da Capo Press, 2006.

Reilly, Patricia Lynn. *A God Who Looks Like Me*. New York: Ballantine Books, 1996.

Reynolds, Jonathan. *Learning to Listen Yoga & Meditation Collective*, www.ayogisway.com and www.learningtolisten.info (Sanskrit interpretations), 2011.

Rupp, Joyce. *Prayers to Sophia*. Notre Dame, IN: Ava Maria Press, 2010.

Steindl-Rast, David. *A Listening Heart: The Art of Contemplative Living*. Chestnut Ridge, NY: The Crossroad Publishing Company, 1983.

Webber, Jerry. *Sometimes an Unknown Path: 40 Psalms-Prayers in Contemporary Voice*. Houston: The Center for Christian Spirituality, 2009.

Webber, Jerry. *Fingerprints on Every Moment*. Houston: The Center for Christian Spirituality, 2010.

Yee, Rodney and Zolotow, Nina. *Yoga: The Poetry of the Body*. New York: St. Martin's Griffin, 2002.

The Yogaphile. *Mudras in Christian Imagery*. http://theyogaphile.blogspot.com/2007/03/mudras-in-christian-imagery.html, 2007.

SCRIPTURE REFERENCES

The Inclusive Bible: The First Egalitarian Translation © 2007. Sheed & Ward.

The Message. Copyright © 1993, 1994, 1995, 1996, 2000, 2001, 2002. Used by permission of NavPress Publishing Group.

The Holy Bible, New International Version®, NIV® Copyright © 1973, 1978, 1984, 2011 by Biblica, Inc.™ Used by permission. All rights reserved worldwide.

The Holy Bible, King James Version. New York: American Bible Society: 1999.

Notes of Namaste

EVERYONE INCLUDED HERE HAS, INDEED, SEEN THE LIGHT IN ME, AND HONORED IT BY ENCOURAGING ME TO SHARE IT.

Namaste to Granny for being a touchstone whose very existence assured me that somehow I too could meld my feminism with my faith. You are missed every day.

And to my parents for the millions of gestures that helped mold me into the person I am. I'll never forget Mom's reminder that "what's on the inside is more important than what's on the outside," while I aspire to live by the optimism contained in Daddy's favorite axiom, "I don't see why not."

To my forever friend, Kim Babineaux, for believing, even before I could write a complete sentence, that we'd walk into a bookstore one day and see my words on the shelf.

To my soul sister, Patty Pinckney, who's tethered to my heart even when she's thousands of miles away. I love that I led you to yoga, and you led me to contemplative spirituality.

To my writing partner and encourager, Jessica Martin-Webber. Our curry lunches fed me in so many ways. I can't wait to sit across from each other with our hard-won books in hand.

To Kim Burt, Lisa Seay and Kelly Hall for riding the roller coaster with me. I look forward to seeing where the journey takes us all. Click...click...click

To Beth Stanley for being a truly wise woman in my life. You are what Sophia would look like in human form.

To Soozin for reminding me that religion isn't the same as spirituality. Your example helped me find the courage to embrace Sophia and share her with others.

To Jeanie Ross for always having a plan that provided hours of testosterone-infused fun for Jack while I cranked out edits.

To Shelby Nielsen for countless impromptu dinners—at your house and mine—while the kids romped and stomped. Many days ours was the only conversation I had outside my own head!

To my sisters, Suzanne, Angie and Sally, who know now that I am not an angel but love me anyway. Angie, your ability to translate my vision into cover art was such a blessing.

To Selise Stewart, whose sophic voice has guided me in my yoga practice on and off the mat. I feel privileged to have called you teacher for more than a decade.

To my publisher and editor Lucy Chambers, a kindred spirit who believed in my book enough to take it on while it was still being birthed. Your exquisite editing and wise questions over breakfast helped shape this book and enabled me to claim my own authority.

To Ellen Cregan and Marla Garcia, who stuck with my flailing attempts to articulate the face of this book until we arrived at a cover that made all of our hearts sing.

To Laura Sheinkopf, who cared enough to help me bring my truest voice to the introduction before heeding the call to return to her rabbinical roots, and to Eva Freeburn who brought her passion to the book's promotion.

To everyone at the "coffice" who asked about the book, encouraged me when I felt stuck, and bought me the occasional cup of coffee while I squirreled away, writing in my purple velvet comfy chair.

To Andie and Jack for helping around the house so I could focus on writing, and for giving me plenty of reasons to take a break from the computer and kick a ball or take a walk together. Playing with you is where life really happens.

To Greg for reading drafts, printing copies, and for paying the Starbucks bill without complaint. Thank you for making space for me to tell this story, and for stoking the fire of my dream when it flickered. I couldn't have done it without your unwavering support.

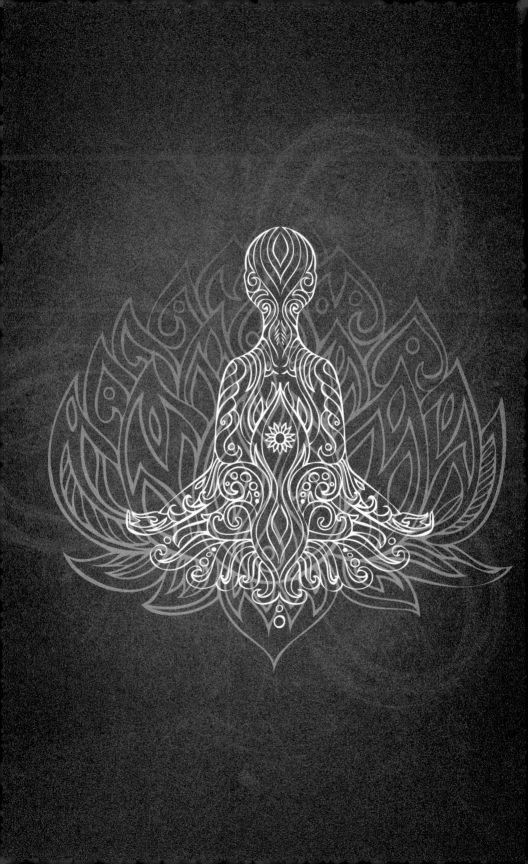